Healthy pregnancy from A to Z :
an expectant parent's guide to wellness

Pregnancy
is a grand adventure
that is about to begin.

Dr Irina Webster

Publisher:
Inspiring Publishers
PO. Box 159, Calwell, ACT Australia 2905
Email: publishaspg@gmail.com
http://www.inspiringpublishers.com

National Library of Australia Cataloguing-in-Publication entry

Author: Webster, Irina

Title: **Healthy pregnancy from A to Z :**
    an expectant parent's guide to wellness/Dr Irina Webster

Subjects: Pregnancy–Health aspects.
Pregnancy–Nutritional aspects.
Prenatal care.

ISBN: 9781925152210 (pbk)

Dewey Number: 618.24

TABLE OF CONTENTS

ABOUT THE AUTHOR

Dr Irina Webster is a medical doctor with a degree in Women and Children's Health. She is a healer and a medical intuitive.

Also by Dr Irina Webster:

Courses and Professional Trainings:

'How to Become a Medical Intuitive and an Intuitive Healer'– professional development training for health professionals and caregivers. This certified 12-month course teaches you how to start practicing intuitive healing and medical intuition on a professional level. **For more information visit** www.intuitive-healing-power.com

CDs

1. **Overcome Stress Naturally with Intuitive Healing.**
   Positive thinking alone is not enough to turn your life around. You must implement strategies to change your emotions from negative and agitated to loving and calming. This will help you create peace in your own heart. Only then you can be free from stress and healed from inside out.

   This CD will help you to overcome stress naturally using your own intuitive healing power. Step by step you will be guided to heal yourself.

2. **Freedom from Pain Using the Intuitive Healing Technique.**
This CD will assist you to activate your own intuitive healing ability and help to relieve pain naturally.

You will also find the meaning of the pain in your life. With the help of this guided meditation you will be able to tune in your body and get to the spot where you experience pain. You will be guided to clean out the blockages and the densities from the place of pain. You will also be guided to heal negative emotions and create more joy, happiness and pleasure in your life.

3. **Body Scan Meditation with Intuitive Healing.**
The purpose of body scan meditation is to study the entire body; part by part. It's like going through your whole body with an x-ray machine checking it organ by organ, muscle by muscle, and bone by bone. This type of x-ray is actually your attention, your mind and your energy.

Body scan meditation helps you experience your body sensations; acknowledge them, tune into them and understand them. It gives you the ability to listen to your body's messages. It allows you to heal, relax and rejuvenate the body parts that require healing.

Step by step you'll be guided to explore your body.

4. **Progressive Muscle Relaxation with Intuitive Healing.**
Progressive relaxation helps you control the state of tension in your muscles. It involves tensing specific muscle groups and then relaxing them to create awareness of tension and relaxation. It is called progressive because it goes through all major muscle groups in the body, relaxing them one at a time, and eventually leads to total muscle relaxation.

Long standing, unreleased muscle tension allows toxic chemicals to grow inside your muscles. This eventually leads to a toxic body and even illness. With this particular meditation you will be able to release all tension and eliminate the toxicity from your body.

Step by step you'll be guided to relax and experience a joyful and loving state.

5. **Create Perfect Health by Activating your Intuitive Healing Power.**

This recording has been designed in order to help you heal, revitalize and restore your energy. You don't have to be unwell to activate your own intuitive healing power. You can use it to prevent illness and to protect yourself from negative energy. It will also help you experience more joy and happiness in your life.

These CDs can be purchased on www.dririnawebster.com

Books

1. **Healthy Pregnancy from A to Z. An Expectant Parent's Guide to Wellness.**
This book is a deep exploration of the most important question **"How to be Healthy during Pregnancy?"** And it shows you a way to parental health and wellbeing while expecting a child.

After reading this book you will discover:
- 5 Healthy Pregnancy Principles.
- The healthiest things to do each month during pregnancy.
- Your baby's development, what they can do and what they can sense each week throughout the duration of pregnancy.
- 21 Best pregnancy foods.
- How to maintain your sex life during pregnancy.
- 7 Healing meditation techniques for pregnancy.
- Special exercise complexes during pregnancy.
- Beneficial yoga poses for different stages of pregnancy.
- 13 Ways to bond with your unborn child.
- The safe herbal remedies to heal pregnancy complaints.
- Natural ways to keep your skin, hair and teeth beautiful during pregnancy.
- How to love your pregnant body.
- Several techniques on self-massage to heal and rejuvenate you during pregnancy.

- How a father-to-be can be a loving partner and a caring dad.
- How to quit your bad habits during pregnancy.
- How music can benefit your pregnancy and what kind of music you should avoid when expecting.
- Steps to ensure a healthy birth and fast, natural recovery. www.inspiringbookshop.com

2. **Secrets to Getting Pregnant. You Can Overcome Infertility.**
This book is rich in practical information and effective strategies on how to get pregnant if you have difficulties conceiving. When you read the book you'll discover:
   - 9 methods to help you get pregnant faster without pain, side effects or discomfort.
   - Specific ways to fall pregnant in older women.
   - Specific ways to get pregnant in cases of "unexplained infertility".
   - A way to a harmonious life as a woman, a wife, and as a mother using the energy of your own cycles. You'll learn to use the cycle's energy instead of letting this energy dominate you.
   - Natural ways to improve your health as a woman in order to get pregnant.
   - A unique way to balance your conscious and subconscious minds, preparing them for motherhood and for attracting a child into your life.
   - How to combine conventional and alternative methods of infertility treatment for best result possible – having a baby.
   - How to know and use your body signs in order to know the exact time to conceive. www.youcanovercomeinfertility.com

3. **Mom Please Help. Anorexia-Bulimia Positive Energy Treatment.**
This book shows you a step-by-step approach to treat eating disorders at home. It contains two parts: one for adults and one for under 18s.
www.mom-please-help.com

4. **Cure Your Eating Disorder: 5 Step Program to Change Your Brain. Neuroplasticity Approach.**

This book shows you a 5 Step Neuroplasticity approach to treat eating disorders.

www.eating-disorders-books.com

Home Treatment Audio Program
Bulimia Home Treatment Program.

Discover the powerful Bulimia home treatment program based on self-directed *neuroplasticity*. Obsessive thoughts, body sensations and subconscious blockages that make you act out your bulimic urges can be stopped with the Power of Neuroplasticity.

www.bulimia-cure.com

Please visit
www.dririnawebster.com
www.intuitive-healing-power.com
www.womenhealthsite.com

INTRODUCTION

Before you were conceived I wanted you. Before you were born I loved you. Before you were here an hour I would die for you. This is the miracle of Mother's Love.
– Maureen Hawkins

Pregnancy brings about great joy and excitement as well as anxiety and concerns. From the time of considering becoming pregnant to the time of having the baby, parents should desire to stay healthy and strong because their health means the health of their baby too. The question 'how to be healthy during pregnancy' has always been one of the most important questions to be asked in a woman's life.

This book is a guide on how to have a healthy pregnancy by discovering and connecting to the natural healing forces inside all of us.

We are the keepers of our own health. We have the power to heal, preserve and restore our health. Many women notice that during pregnancy the natural healing forces inside the body become more evident. Internal awareness heightens. This awareness can help you stay healthy throughout pregnancy and beyond.

Even though everyone has a different background and medical history, it is possible to make any pregnancy the healthiest you possibly can. It is all in your own hands.

Just relying on somebody else (doctors, midwives and other health professionals) to provide you with a healthy pregnancy without any activity by yourself and working on your own well-being is a big mistake. To experience good health during pregnancy you need to make a commitment and implement lots of action plans towards being healthy.

It does not mean blaming yourself (or somebody else) for feeling unwell. On the contrary, it means accepting your experiences and being grateful for who you're and the life you have. It also means loving your pregnant body and knowing it, understanding the signs of what your body needs.

The following principles are the bedrock on which a healthy pregnancy can be built. Read them and think where you're at with each point:

Healthy Pregnancy Principles:

1. **In order to have a healthy pregnancy, you need to commit to making your health and the health of your baby a priority.** You need to commit to such things as:
   - Organising your antenatal care early.
   - Eating well.
   - Being careful with food hygiene.
   - Taking folic acid supplements.
   - Exercising regularly.
   - Doing pelvic floor exercises daily.
   - Quitting smoking and alcohol.
   - Cutting back on caffeine.
   - Getting more rest and relaxation.
     And probably much more…

2. **You should be in touch with your feelings and listen to your body**. Many women spend much of their time thinking and rationalizing rather than "feeling". But our feelings

are the signs and language of our body. By ignoring and dismissing their feelings, women are often ignoring their body's needs. You should be able to recognise when you need to rest, play, have fun, and work. Your body is constantly talking to you through feelings, sensations, dreams and mental pictures. You must pay attention to these. Regular meditation can help you to stay in touch with your feelings, accept them and learn from them.

3. **Bring conscious awareness to your body.**

   This can be done by practicing *conscious breathing and conscious eating*. Whatever you do during the day be aware of your breath as much as you can. Don't let your mind wander, just feel the air moving in and out of your body. When you eat, be consciously aware of what you eat, how fast you eat and fully enjoy the taste of every bite. As you regularly practice conscious breathing and conscious eating you become more aware of your organs and of your baby in the womb. Regular meditation can help you bring conscious awareness to your body.

4. **Move your body and exercise**.

   Regular physical activity will help you feel better, enjoy your body, have more energy, detoxify and heal. Also, considering the fact that *babies can learn while in the womb*, you actually teach your child to exercise and stay healthy *even before birth*. Plan an exercise program that you will enjoy, such as walking, jogging, swimming, dancing, yoga, regular stretching etc. In this book we describe many exercise regimes that you can do at home when pregnant.

5. **Create the biochemistry of gratitude.**

   The attitude of gratitude creates grateful feelings. Grateful feelings, continuously reinforced by positive thoughts and actions will change the biochemistry of your body to the very best. *Attitude of gratitude can actually make you healthy and heal wounds.* Even if you have problems, be grateful for them as overcoming them is your blessing.

Pregnancy is a time of questions?

During pregnancy it is natural, that you have questions. All women have, even the most experienced mothers. Even women-doctors have questions when they become pregnant.

What is healthy to eat? What are the best pregnancy foods?

What is a healthy life style during pregnancy?

What you must avoid while pregnant?

What is a healthy pregnancy weight?

How to develop healthy habits and stop bad ones?

What is a healthy bump size during different stages of pregnancy? And what about the bump shape?

How is the baby feeling inside?

What does the baby look like at current point in time?

What are the safe things to do while pregnant and what are not?

Minor worries can become major fears if you don't know the answers. In this book we go through the whole pregnancy week by week, month by month. You'll see and learn what your baby is like each week and what healthy things you can do during the duration of your pregnancy.

It is all about self-healing during pregnancy, listening to your body and being in tune with yourself and your baby.

> *"Natural forces within us are the true healers of disease."*
> – Hippocrates, The father of Medicine.

CHAPTER 1

Preparing for a Healthy Pregnancy

Why it is important to prepare yourself for pregnancy?

It is worth your time and effort to start preparing yourself for pregnancy at least 1-3 months ahead. Your body and mind will go through many changes during pregnancy, so the stronger you get before it - the more comfortable you will be during your pregnancy.

The preparation for a healthy pregnancy includes 4 important parts.

1. Your beliefs and attitudes.
2. Your knowledge about pregnancy and health.
3. Your body.
4. Your emotions.

Your pre-pregnancy beliefs and attitudes.

It is no secret that your personal believes and attitudes affect your health and fertility. A growing body of scientific evidence suggests that faith can bring us good health. People who attend religious services or regularly practice a form of spirituality are healthier and have a lower risk of illnesses than people who don't have a nurturing spiritual path. People who believe in a loving God recover and heal much faster than those who believe in a punitive God.

In regards to getting pregnant it is the same: your reproductive system has eyes and ears. It takes in everything. The beliefs you and your partner convey about your fertility can directly affect your ability to conceive and have a healthy child.

> **Advice:** *When trying to conceive, adopt a loving attitude. Beware of negative messages. Do all things with love. Create a loving energy field around yourself.*

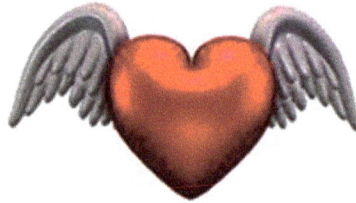

What do you know about pregnancy and health?

Knowledge is power. The more you know about pregnancy the easier it is for you to be in control of your reproductive function. Becoming conscious of your body structure will help complete your self-image and bring awareness to your body.

The more intimately you know the physical make up of your reproductive organs and all the organs which participate in pregnancy, the more successful your health-intervention will be.

Knowing the anatomy of the body and its systems (at least basic) can help you visualise the natural physiological processes when you practice self-healing.

For instance, if you're over 35 and you have problems with ovulation, being able to visualize the healthy ovulation process can help you to achieve a successful pregnancy. There are two focal points that you can tune into by knowing the natural ovula¬tion process of your body.

1st focal point: Your hypothalamus (in the brain) stimulates your pituitary glands which send out follicle-stimulating hormone (FSH).

2nd focal point: Then your ovaries, stimulated by FSH release an egg which travels down the fallopian tube for fertilization.

If you sit quietly and visualise this process and that everything is working properly, then you enhance the chances of getting pregnant. This is true for any problem you may encounter during pregnancy.

You can do the same things (visualising of a healthy process) for any problems you might experience before, during or after pregnancy.

> **Advice:** *learn a bit of simple anatomy concerning your body and some basic physiology of the processes related to pregnancy can help.*

What should you learn?

- Structure of the reproductive organs.
- Simple mechanics of conception.
- Hormones that play a role in conception and pregnancy.

All this knowledge will make you more powerful and help you to become prepared for a healthy pregnancy. Knowledge is really power.

Note:

If you are over 35, or have had at least 3 miscarriages in the past, or already have a child with a birth defect, or have a complicated medical history in the family, you may consider **genetic testing.** You can ask your doctor about that if you are worried.

Getting ready for Pregnancy.

Your body.

Your body should be strong enough to carry a child and be ready to cope with the many changes pregnancy brings.

This preparation includes: *healthy eating, physical exercise and avoiding environmental dangers (chemicals, pollution, radiation etc.).*

The healthy eating requirements for pre-pregnant women are the same as healthy eating for most people of the same age, gender, and physical activity level. But there are two exceptions: these are iron and folate/folic acid.

Pre-pregnancy diet should include:

- *Take folic acid at least 400 micrograms (mcg) daily. You will also find it in fortified breakfast cereals; citrus fruits and juices; dried peas and beans; and green leafy vegetables such as spinach, collard and turnip greens, and broccoli.*

Folic acid helps a baby's neural tube (the part of the embryo that becomes the brain and spinal cord) develop properly. It is critical to start taking it before conception and to continue taking it through to the third month of pregnancy when the baby's neural tube is developing. This can help to prevent birth defects in the spine and the skull of your baby.

Folic acid also plays an important role in regulating moods, has antidepressant properties, and strengthens your heart and metabolism.

- Eat foods high in iron (meat, fish, and poultry) as well as foods that facilitate iron absorption, such as vitamin C-rich foods like oranges, orange juice, cantaloupe, strawberries, and grapefruit. Also vegetables such as broccoli, brussel sprouts, tomato, tomato juice, potatoes, and green and red peppers.

Iron is also very important during pregnancy as it prevents anaemia, a condition in which the body isn't able to produce enough healthy red blood cells. Developing babies need a high level of red blood cells in order to receive enough oxygen. Anaemia in the mother can be passed on to her baby.

- Eat a variety of fruits and vegetables, preferably fresh, but canned and frozen can be ok too. The most important vegetables are: dark green veggies, such as broccoli, kale, and other dark leafy greens; orange veggies, such as carrots, sweet potatoes, pumpkin, and winter squash; beans and peas such as pinto beans, kidney beans, black beans, garbanzo beans (chick peas), split peas, and lentils.

- Eat your calcium-rich foods also. Milk and dairy products are great sources of calcium. 3 cups of low-fat or fat-free milk or an equivalent amount of low-fat yogurt and/or low-fat cheese (30 g of cheese equals 1 cup of milk) can cover your daily requirements of calcium. If you don't or can't consume milk, choose lactose-free milk products and/or calcium-fortified foods and beverages. The recommended daily allowance is 1,000 mg. For Vegans, consume calcium rich plants (almonds, broccoli, spring greens, kale, currants, oranges, figs, soy milk, tahini, tofu and wholemeal bread).

- Whole-grains. Eat at least 80-85 g of whole-grain cereals, breads, crackers, rice, or pasta every day. This amount is equal to 1 slice of bread, 1 cup of breakfast cereal, or ½ cup of cooked rice or pasta.

- *Go lean with protein. Choose lean meats and poultry. Bake it, broil it, or grill it. Also vary your protein choices with more fish, beans, peas, nuts, and seeds.*
- *Eat different nuts. About 100-140 g a week of nuts is a healthy addition to any diet – unless you're allergic to them.*
- *Limit your consumption of fats, salt, and sugars.*

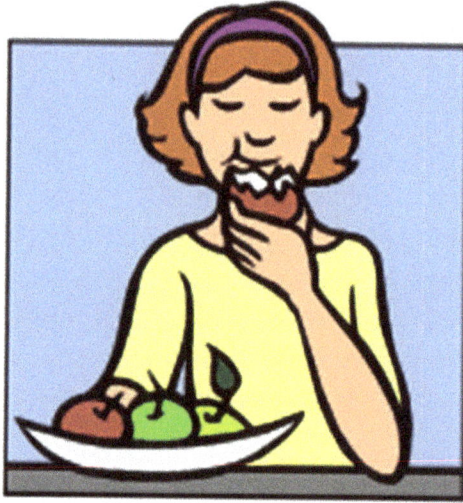

Pre-pregnancy exercise is the same as any healthy person of your age and weight. Exercise 30-40 min at least 3-4 times a week for general wellbeing. If you need to lose weight – exercise at least 30 min every day. Any physical activity is good but it is important to be an intensive activity (until you really sweat) to make you lose weight.

There are three types of activities you can do:

1. *Cardiovascular exercise (aerobic training)* includes walking, running, cycling, swimming, aerobic dancing.
   For health and to strengthen your heart, lungs and immune system; 30 minutes a day is best, but at least 20 minutes a day three to five times a week is okay. Studies show

that three 10-minute sessions a day are as good as one 30-minute workout.

To lose weight, do at least 40 to 60 minutes of continuous exercise (basically until you sweat properly) three or more times a week.

For endurance, to be prepared for labour and keeping up after the baby is born, 30 minutes a day is best or at least 20 minutes a day three to five times a week.

2. *Strength training (anaerobic)* includes lifting free weights, using resistance machines, doing isometrics. Aqua aerobics is good to do for resistance work as the water offers support plus resistance. Work all your major muscle groups twice a week. These activities strengthen your bones and muscles, and they boost your metabolism (increase the number of calories you burn).

3. *Flexibility training (stretching, doing yoga or tai chi)*. Do this every day for 10-20 minutes. These exercises keep you flexible, reduce your risk of injuries, and improve how you feel in general.

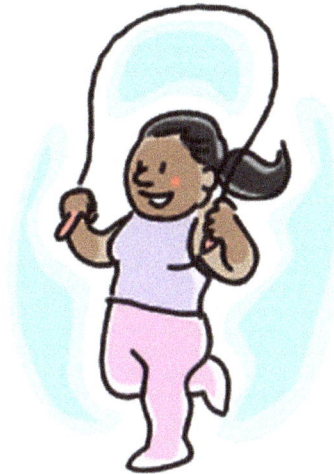

Avoiding environmental dangers before pregnancy:

- It is important to avoid contact with pesticides and be aware of chemicals you use at home e.g. for cleaning and washing. Try to use natural stuff for cleaning purposes such as soda, vinegar and different herbs. Avoid hair dyes and hair sprays; use herbal solutions instead. Avoid radiation and use gloves when changing the cat litter. Toxo plasmosis is a parasite transmitted to humans by contact with faeces from an infected cat and could cause problems.

- Be careful about eating certain fish, including shark, swordfish, king mackerel and tilefish. Sometimes these fish contain mercury that can affect fertility and the foetus.

- Reduce or avoid consumption of caffeine, alcohol and nicotine.

Your pre-pregnancy emotions.

Your emotions are very important and they affect fertility in many ways. Some women do not get pregnant because in their hearts they really do not want to; they are afraid of the demands a child will make on them. This internal conflict over birthing or the restrictions that children may bring affects fertility in a negative way. Scientific studies have suggested an association between infertility and ambivalence towards pregnancy and children.

The relationships between partners who can't get pregnant have also been studied. Many of the women in these studies had an actual aversion to intercourse; they had low levels of orgasm when they do have intercourse, and they felt a marked sexual disharmony in their partnership. When these women found more suitable partners, however, they became fertile.

The important thing here is that the same small part of the brain the hypothalamus, controls stress and emotions as well as fertility and sex drive.

The advice here is not to look for another partner but reassess your deep emotions that are inside your heart regarding childbirth and your intimate relationship.

The questions below can help you become clearer on how you really feel:

1. As a child, did you hear negative words/stories about menstruation, pregnancy or childbirth from your parents, grandparents, aunts or uncles?
2. What did you hear about your mother's pregnancy with you and your birth? From which parent? Do the stories differ between your mother and father? With what kind of emotions were these stories told to you? Were the stories told with love and caring, or ambivalence, indifference, anger or aversion?
3. In your opinion, were children valued by your mother, father, grandparents and siblings? Do you feel that you were valued and how?
4. How does your family view working women and motherhood?
5. Are many of your major life decisions based upon whether your parents would approve?
7. Why do you want to have a baby? Or why don't you?

When you analyse your responses you may see some family issues that can affect your fertility and pregnancy.

Just being aware of where your negative feelings about pregnancy come from will provide you with the ability to attach new meanings to things and change them.

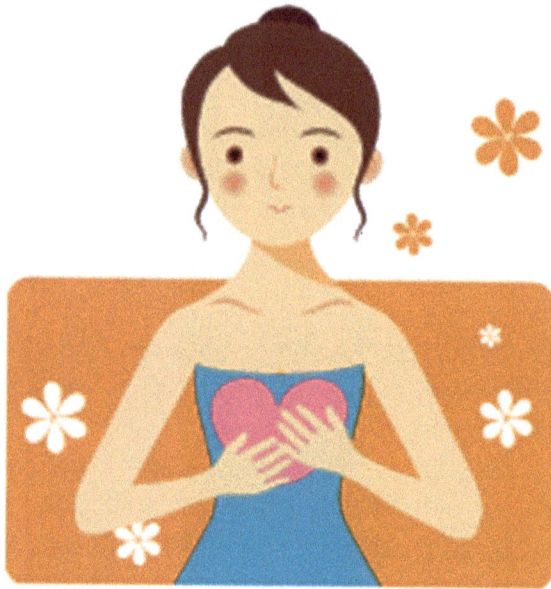

Positive attitude to motherhood.

Having positive emotions about motherhood is also important because maternal emotions and feelings can leave a permanent mark on a child's personality. It is proven now that while in uterus, a child can see, hear, taste, and on a primitive level even learn. Most importantly he can feel, although not with an adult complexity, but feel nonetheless. The main source of a baby's feelings is the child's pregnant mother.

This doesn't mean that every single worry or anxiety of a woman will damage the child. But deep persistent patterns of maternal emotions will play a role in shaping the child's personality and health.

The father's feelings about pregnancy are equally important. That's why both parents should reassess their intimate feelings about child baring and parenthood.

> **Advice:** *Start doing regular meditation. Meditation is a great way to heal yourself from any negative emotions and former conditioning, including parental. It also increases your awareness which gives you more control over your own body. You'll become more in tune with all the processes inside including ovulation, conception and the baby.*

Other things you should check out before pregnancy.

Medications.

If you take any medications (including all prescription, over-the-counter, and alternative remedies including herbs) you should review them with your doctor before pregnancy. Some medicines can cause serious birth defects and miscarriage.

Dental care.

The health of your teeth and gums can affect the growth and development of the foetus.

It is important to brush and floss your teeth to prevent gingivitis; a gum disease. Studies show that gum disease and oral infections can increase your risk for premature birth and low birth weight babies from either preterm labour or premature rupture of the membranes (your water breaks early).

Visit your dentist while preparing to get pregnant for a check up.

Shettles's system – How to increase the odds of having a boy or a girl in your favour.

This is the fun part of getting pregnant; you never know which sex the baby will be. Some couples happily accept whatever comes along, a boy or a girl. But for some it is important to have a child of a particular sex. Although there is no absolute certainty method of having a boy or a girl, there is a system which allows you to increase your chances of have a child of a particular sex.

Following the Shettles's system is a great fun so you will not lose anything by trying it out.

Using this system is free; it absolutely does not cost you any money, only your determination and desire. It is called Shettles's system after Dr Shettles who is one of the most influential fertility experts of the last 50 years and often considered as the father of IVF.

Many people say that at best, this system increases the chances of a child of a particular sex from 50% to 75%. It is definitely NOT a guarantee of success, but it is currently the most well-known method for influencing gender without the use of medical procedures.

The method is based on the premise that men produce two types of sperm, the X (female) and Y (male). The Y sperms are smaller and more delicate, but faster, than the X sperms which are bigger, tougher and slower. The system is based on providing an environment which is more likely to help the type of sperm that matches your preference to get to the egg first.

There are six basic recommendations to follow:

1) Timing - the most critical aspect of the Shettle's method is to time when you have intercourse. The closer to ovulation that you have sex, the better your chances of having a boy, because ovulation provides the most optimal time for conceiving, and male sperm are faster. If you have intercourse about 3 days prior to ovulation, you may maximize the chances for the slower but tougher female sperm, which are able to survive until the egg appears.

2) The pH of the woman's vagina is also important. A more alkaline environment is generally favourable to fertility and, therefore, favours the quicker, but more delicate, male sperm. For a girl, a douche of very diluted water and vinegar is done just before intercourse. For a boy, a douche of very diluted water and baking soda just before intercourse is indicated.

3) Penetration during intercourse. Intercourse with shallow penetration may favour the conception of a girl, and intercourse with deeper penetration is believed to favour a boy.

4) Orgasms in females produce a hormone which makes their vaginal tract more alkaline and therefore more favourable for boys.

5) A high sperm count favours boys. To increase sperm count, Shettle's method recommends that you abstain from intercourse for up to three to four days before ovulation. Also, men should wear boxers rather than tight underpants.
To reduce the sperm count, men should take a hot bath just before intercourse and couples should have as much intercourse as possible until 3 days before ovulation.

6) Drinking a cup of coffee just prior to intercourse tends to favour a boy.

To sum up all of the above:

To Increase the Chance of Having a Girl:

- Use a vaginal douche, consisting of 20 ml white vinegar in 500 ml of water, ten minutes before having sex.
- Have sex frequently in the seven to ten days before you ovulate.
- Have no sex from one day before ovulation until ten days after ovulation.

- Your partner should ejaculate just inside the vagina, and not deeply inside.
- Your partner should withdraw immediately after ejaculation.
- It is better for the woman not to have an orgasm.

To Increase the Chance of Having a Boy:

- Ten minutes before sex, use a vaginal douche consisting of 5 g of baking soda in 500 mg of water.
- Have no sex from the end of your period until the day ovulation occurs.
- Have sex twice daily from the day of ovulation until four days afterward.
- Your partner should ejaculate deep inside the vagina.
- Your partner should not withdraw immediately after ejaculation.
- It is better for the woman to have an orgasm; ideally just before ejaculation.

Good luck!

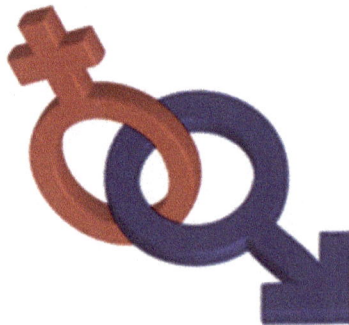

CHAPTER 2

Your First Symptoms of Pregnancy

Conception occurs about 2 weeks before your period is due. This means that you may be more than 3 weeks pregnant and not even know that you're pregnant!

This is important because your baby is most sensitive to harm in the period from two to eight weeks after conception. This is when your baby's facial features and organs, such as the heart and kidneys, begin to form.

Anything that you eat, drink, smoke or are exposed to, can affect your baby during this time. That's why it's the best to start acting as if you're pregnant before you know that you have conceived. That's why preparation for pregnancy is important.

Symptoms of Early Pregnancy?

You may begin to suspect you're pregnant soon after conception, but only if you're extremely well tuned into your body's rhythms. Women who meditate regularly, doing yoga or pursue some spiritual practices are more in tune with their bodies than those who don't practice anything. This is why I recommend you to start practicing meditation before you fall pregnant.

Many women won't experience any noticeable early pregnancy symptoms until the fertilized egg attaches itself to the uterine wall, several days after conception. Some may notice no signs of pregnancy at all and begin to wonder, "Am I pregnant?" only when they miss a period.

There are some first signs of impending motherhood. You may experience all, some, or none of these symptoms during the early stages of your pregnancy:

1) **Tender swollen breasts:** Your breasts may provide one of the first symptoms of pregnancy. As early as two weeks after conception, hormonal changes may make your breasts tender, tingly or sore. Or your breasts may feel fuller and heavier. A tingling sensation will be felt in the nipples. Once your body grows accustomed to the hormone surge, the pain will subside.

2) **Darkening of your areolas:** This can happen as early as a week or two after conception. Some women may notice bumps (resembling goose-bumps) pop up on the perimeter of their areolas. These are called Montgomery tubercles. They provide lubrication to your nipples, when you start feeding the baby. But, this may also signal a hormonal imbalance that is unrelated to pregnancy or be a left-over effect from a previous pregnancy. It can even be related to the consumption of oral contraceptive pills.

3) **Frequent urination:** This is mainly because the blood flow to a woman's kidneys increases by up to 35 to 60% due to hormonal changes. The extra blood flow makes her kidneys produce up to 25% more urine soon after conception.

4) **Dark patches on forehead and cheeks:** These patches are caused by hormonal changes that affect the pigment cells in the skin; they are called 'chloasma'. This can also happen

as a side-effect of the contraceptive pills. The navel and a line down the centre of the woman's belly may also darken.

5) **Food cravings:** Food cravings can sometimes be a sign of pregnancy. Don't rely on them as a sure symptom; it may be all in your head, or even a sign that your body is low on a particular nutrient. But if the cravings are accompanied by some of the other symptoms on this list, the chances are you're pregnant.

6) **Implantation bleeding or cramping:** You may experience implantation spotting, a slight staining of a pink or brown colour, as well as some cramping about eight days after ovulation. You might also see some spotting around the time you expect your period; this is caused by the egg burrowing into the endometrial lining. Some women have increased vaginal discharge in early in pregnancy.

7) **Fatigue:** High levels of the hormone progesterone can make you feel tired; as if you've run a marathon, when all you've done is to put in a day at the office. Tiredness is a hallmark of early pregnancy, though probably not a sure symptom on its own.

8) **Morning sickness:** You may begin feeling nauseated and queasy as early as a couple of days after conception. But often, morning sickness begins a few weeks after conception. Some women don't have it at all. Nausea can occur any time: morning, evening or even at night. You may also notice that your sense of taste changes. Some women say they have a metallic taste in their mouth, others that they cannot stand the taste of coffee, tea or a food they usually like.

9) **Your basal body temperature stays high:** You will notice this only if you've been charting your basal body temperature.

If your basal body temperature has stayed above the cover line for 18 days in a row, you're probably pregnant.

Basal body temperature is your temperature taken the first thing in the morning before you get up, usually about 6 a.m. It is important to keep taking it at the same time. The temperature can be taken orally, vaginally or rectally – just stay with the same method for the entire cycle.

10) **Excessive salivation:** Excessive salivation can happen at around 6 week gestation as a result of changing hormone levels. Excessive saliva may happen sporadically during periods of rapid hormonal fluctuation like during the first and third trimesters.

11) **Headaches** in early pregnancy also are caused by hormonal changes, but they may also be due to the normal increase in blood volume circulating in the woman's system during pregnancy.

12) **Bloating and constipation** are common in the first trimester. It happens because the hormone progesterone slows the movement or 'motility' of the gut.

Pregnancy Confirmation with Medical Tests.

To confirm your pregnancy you can use two kinds of tests:

- A blood test at a doctor's office, **5-7 days** after conception.
- A home pregnancy test, **10 days** after you think you may have become pregnant.

All pregnancy tests measure the amount *of human chorionic gonadotropin (hCG),* the pregnancy hormone in your body.

The blood test for pregnancy measures the amount of hCG in your bloodstream. Blood tests can measure much smaller amounts of the hormone, and so can detect pregnancy earlier than urine tests, usually about 5-7 days after ovulation. However, these are only available through your doctor who is unlikely to offer one unless you have pressing medical reasons to know quickly whether or not you are pregnant. This test is 99% accurate.

Home pregnancy tests are less accurate compare to blood test. To increase their accuracy, use the first urine of the day; hCG is most easily detected then, follow the instructions carefully, and recheck your test results the next morning and again in a week unless your period has started.

Why Incorrect Results may Occur?
You may get a false-positive or false-negative result.

Possible Causes of False-Positives:
- Using an unclean urine collection cup.
- Using an old or damaged kit.
- Having an impure urine sample.
- Taking certain prescription drugs.

Possible Causes of a False-Negative Result:
- Taking the test too early.
- Performing the test later than 15 minutes after collecting the urine sample.

Obstetric Ultrasound
Ultrasound can confirm the pregnancy too, but it is usually performed for medical reasons. Talk to your doctor if you need to have one.

There are two ways to perform the test: Trans abdominal; through an Abdomen ultrasound or Vaginal ultrasound. You may be instructed to drink up to six glasses of water and avoid urinating until the procedure is completed for Trans abdominal ultrasound. Vaginal ultrasound is performed on empty bladder.

Calculation of Delivery Date.

Congratulations again!!!! You are definitely pregnant. Now, you probably would like to know when the baby is due. You need to prepare yourself because you are a **mother-to-be.**

There is a simple formula to calculate the approximate delivery date. You can do it yourself.

Just add on 7 days to when the last period started and then add 9 months; e.g. if the last period started on 5th January 2013 (05.01.13), then the baby will be due on 12th October 2013 (12.10.13). The calculation is shown again in the example below:

First day of last period = 05. 01. 13
+ 7 days = 12. 01. 13
+ 9 months = 12. 10. 13

A standard pregnancy lasts 40 weeks (280 days) from the beginning of the last period, but only 38 weeks from conception, because a woman ovulates two weeks after her period starts.

Pregnancy is counted from the day of the mother's last menstrual period. This means that, at conception, the unborn child is considered to be two weeks old.

Only 5% of women deliver their babies on their projected due date, so this date should only be used as an estimate, it is not an exact calculation.

Healthy things to do when you find out you're pregnant.

What are the most important things to do when you find out that you are pregnant?

Answer: Taking care of yourself by nurturing yourself and the baby. Here are some recommendations:

1. *Choose a doctor/specialist you want to see during your pregnancy.*

Choosing the right doctor is an important decision. There are several kinds of practitioners to choose from:

- Obstetricians are doctors who specialize in the care of women during pregnancy and childbirth.
- Family practice doctors are doctors with training in all aspects of health care for every member of the family.
- Certified midwifes are registered nurses with advanced, specialized training in taking care of pregnant women and delivering babies.
- Maternalfoetal medicine specialists are obstetrician with special training in the care of women who have high-risk pregnancies. You can be referred to this practitioner if you have risk-factors in your medical history or pregnancy complications.

It's easy to feel overwhelmed by the choice, but with a little research, you should be able to find the person you like and trust.

The qualities to look for in a health care practitioner are:

- Look for someone who takes time to listen to you, who pays attention and lets you fully explain your concerns. Good eye contact is a good sign that a doctor is attentive and careful.
- Choose a technically qualified practitioner and who won't get offended if you ask for a second opinion.
- Choose someone who honours your feelings, intuitions and thoughts about your pregnancy, health and the baby.
- Avoid those who make you feel guilty or foolish for expressing yourself and asking questions, who approach you with a demeaning "holier than thou" attitude and who don't return phone calls or rush you through the visit.

The relationship with your doctor should be healing. You must feel good visiting him/her and the energy exchange during the visit must be very positive. Deep healing depends upon the chemistry and respect you share with your caregiver. Choose them wisely.

2. **Stop drinking and smoking.**

   There are no safe amounts of alcohol or nicotine during pregnancy. Any even very small amounts of these substances can cause damage to the baby.

   Embracing spirituality is a great way to stop any addictions including addictions to alcohol and nicotine. If you start regular meditation, it can help you to overcome the troublesome urges to drink and/or smoke.

3. **Reduce caffeine.**

   Caffeine is a stimulant and a diuretic. Because caffeine is a stimulant, it increases your blood pressure and heart rate, both of which are not recommended during pregnancy. Caffeine also increases the frequency of urination. This causes reduction in your body fluid levels and can lead to dehydration.

   Caffeine crosses the placenta to your baby. Any amount of caffeine can also cause changes in your baby's sleep pattern or normal movement pattern in the later stages of pregnancy.

   Caffeine is found in coffee, tea, soft drinks, chocolate, and even some over the counter medications for the relief of headaches. Be aware of what you consume.

   It is recommended for pregnant women to have less than 200 mg of caffeine a day. See how easy you can overdose this safe amount:

1 mug of instant coffee = 100 mg
1 cup of instant coffee = 75 mg
1 cup of brewed coffee = 100 mg to 350 mg,
depending on beans and how it is made
1 cup of tea = 50 mg
1 can of cola = 40 mg
1 can of "energy" drink = 80 mg
1 x 50 g bar of plain chocolate = up to 50 mg
1 x 50 g bar of milk chocolate = up to 25 mg

Remember that the amount of caffeine in coffee and tea can vary widely depending on the quality of the product and the way it is prepared. Just be constantly aware of caffeine consumption and remember to substitute it with decaffeinated coffee, tea or soft drink (non-cola).

4. **Medicines**. Check out with your doctor regarding all the medicines, drugs, complementary and alternative medicines you are using or planning to use. Most drugs are dangerous during pregnancy. Many alternative medicines such as herbs are not safe during pregnancy either. Use the adage "Its better be safe than sorry" approach to all medicines and remedies while pregnant.

5. **Exercise regularly but within your limits**. The best exercise is moderate, enjoyable and something you can do on most days of the week such as walking, swimming or yoga. Avoid overheating in spas and saunas. Always drink plenty of fluids when exercising.

6. **Eat healthy.** Pregnancy creates extra demands for certain nutrients, including iron, calcium, iodine and many vitamins, so make sure your diet is varied and includes adequate amounts of the fruits and vegetables, breads and cereals, dairy foods for calcium, lean meats, chicken and fish for iron.

7. **Practice hygiene and food safety.** Wash your hands, cook dishes properly, wash vegetables and fruit before eating them. Also avoid cold sliced meats, uncooked seafood, soft-serve ice-cream, pre-prepared salads and cheeses such as brie, camembert, feta and ricotta.

8. **Take folate supplements 500 mcg (0.5 mg) daily.** It is best to start taking folate at least two months before you get pregnant. If you haven't taken it before start right now. This will reduce the risk of spinal problems such as spina bifida in your baby. Folate also helps you to stay healthy: it protects your heart, improves your blood, reduces depression and keeps your brain young.

9. **Sun and air exposure.** Regularly get fresh air, spend some time under the sun to make your skin produce Vitamin D which is vital for baby's development.

CHAPTER 3

Pregnancy Week by Week, Month by Month

Feels Fat the last 9 months,
but the joy of becoming a mum lasts forever.

Whether planned or unplanned, pregnancy is one of the most beautiful things that can ever happen in a woman's life. For the next nine months, you will be carrying your baby inside you, nourishing and nurturing it inside your body until baby is ready to come out into the world.

While pregnancy is a beautiful thing, it is also very life-changing. The following nine months will definitely be a rollercoaster ride of mixed emotions and uncomfortable symptoms. You may also notice unfamiliar changes in your body, leading you to ask yourself many questions.

What is happening inside me?

Is my baby okay?

How can I keep him or her safe?

Why am I experiencing these symptoms?

What can I do to feel better?

Not knowing what is happening to your body or your baby can cause worries or anxieties. Arming yourself with lots of information will allow you to take care of your body and your baby better as you prepare yourself for changes that will surely come in the following months.

Month 1 (1st to 4th week)

How Is Your Baby?

The first month of pregnancy is quite different from the following months to come. This is because during the first two weeks of pregnancy, you are considered not even pregnant at all. This may sound confusing at first, but it is important to note that determining the actual time of conception is basically impossible. So the doctor will calculate your due date starting from the first day of your last menstrual cycle.

> **Week 1:** The first week of pregnancy begins with the first day of your menstrual period. You are not pregnant just yet but the countdown to baby begins this week. 'Why is this?' You may ask. Well here is why?
>
> You see, it is known that conception takes place sometime after your period. So it is usually around 14 days after the start of your period, although time can vary depending on the lengths of your cycle and the time you had intercourse. There is no exact science that can work out exactly the moment of conception. But it is easy to remember when your period started and that's why the first day of your period is considered to be the first day of your pregnancy. We use this just for convenience and the ease in calculating conception.
>
> **Week 2:** Remember you are still not technically pregnant yet. The second week is the one right after your men-

struation. During this time, your body prepares for ovulation, which happens right around the end of the week or the beginning of the next. In the beginning of this week your ovarian follicles are maturing until one is destined to become a proper egg. The lining of your uterus is thickening and preparing for the coming implantation. Right around the end of the second week, your ovary releases a single egg cell that travels all the way down the fallopian tube then waits for fertilization.

Week 3: Now you have actually conceived! Fertilization is when your partner's sperm cell penetrates your egg cell, causing pregnancy. Congratulations!!! Out of the 300 million or more sperm released by your partner, only one will fertilise your egg. The conception takes place in the fallopian tube, where the egg has waited from the week before. The gender of your baby is determined by your partner's single successful sperm, which will contain either a male Y chromosome or female X chromosome. As soon as the egg is fertilised, it starts to rapidly divide. The fertilised egg, now called an ovum, starts to move slowly away from the tube and down into the uterus.

Week 4: Implantation has just occurred. The ovum - the fertilised egg settles itself in the lining of your uterus, and this is called implantation. This is when you may first start to suspect you are actually pregnant. At this time, your baby grows from a single cell to a thousand cells blastocyst.

The blastocyst has two different layers of cells: the outer and inner layers. The outer layer forms the placenta, the round and flat organ responsible for transferring food and nutrients to your baby. The inner layer forms the organs and parts of the baby's body. The placenta produces the human chrorionic gonadotropin or hCG – the pregnancy hormone which is detected by pregnancy tests. As the fertilized egg grows, the amniotic fluid fills the sac around it, cushioning the growing embryo right up until birth. Blood cells will begin to develop during the fourth week as well, allowing blood circulation to begin.

The embryo starts its division into three layers, the endoderm, the inner layer, the mesoderm, the middle layer and the ectoderm, the outer layer. The endoderm, the inner layer will develop into the liver, pancreas, gastrointestinal tract, thyroid and the lungs. The mesoderm, the middle layer will develop into the heart, sex organs, muscles, bones, bone marrow and kidneys. The ectoderm, the outer layer will develop into the nervous system, sweat glands, enamel of the teeth, skin, eyes, hair and nails. So, as you can see organ and system development starts at the 4th week of pregnancy.

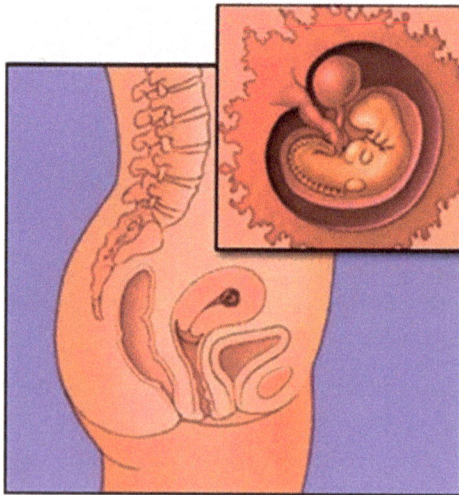

Your baby at the first month.

Your experiences during the 1st month of pregnancy.

Most women will not notice any symptoms or changes in the body during the first two weeks of pregnancy except of the normal pre-menstrual or menstrual symptoms you always have. This is because conception has not happened just yet. During the last two weeks however, you may experience a wide range of physical and emotional changes. These include:

- Implantation bleeding. This may look like a light period but normally it is more like spotting which lasts a day or two.
- Breast tenderness.
- Fatigue, sleepiness during the day.
- Nausea and increased sensitivity to smells.
- More frequent urination than usual.
- Headaches.
- Heartburn.
- Constipation, bloating and flatulence.
- Cramping.
- Slight increase in your body temperature.

Emotionally you may feel irritable, occasional mood swings and increased sensitivity.

Each woman responds differently to the changes that pregnancy brings. This means that you may or may not experience all of these symptoms mentioned above. Still, these physical and emotional changes are very common during the first three months of pregnancy, so you will most likely experience at least one or a couple of them during the first month.

All these symptoms in early pregnancy are due to the production of a pregnancy hormone the *human chorionic gonadotriopin* or hGC. This pregnancy hormone is produced by placenta, a new organ which brings nutrition and oxygen to your baby.

Healthythings to do during the 1st month of pregnancy.

Most of the symptoms in early pregnancy are temporary and will go away in a few months or even earlier. You can take control of some of these symptoms by changing your diet and learning how to relax.

Regarding your diet you should eat small meals throughout the day to prevent hunger pangs and heartburn. At this time you may start to have cravings and food aversions also. It is okay to give into these cravings, but be careful not to eat too much as this may trigger nausea and vomiting. For constipation issues, make sure that you include fibre rich foods in your diet. Some fruits and vegetables are particularly helpful to relief constipation: these are plumbs, apricots, figs, beetroot and cabbage.

Hormone changes in the body may cause you to feel tired and stressed throughout the day. Help yourself feel better by de-stressing through relaxation exercises. Meditation, yoga and breathing techniques are particularly helpful to make you feel better and become more in tune with your body and with the baby.

Meditation, yoga and breathing techniques will help you not just to relieve stress and fatigue but also help to cease some aches and pains associated with pregnancy, make heartburn less noticeable and give you more energy to cope throughout the day.

Healthy and practical things to do in the beginning of pregnancy.

1. **Start a pregnancy journal.** Buy a new notebook and call it "My pregnancy journal". Take a bit of time every day and write down your thoughts and feelings. It is very helpful to write your journal first thing in the morning, when your brain is fresh and is preparing for a new day. Whatever you feel, whatever comes to mind, just jot it down. Nothing is

too petty, too silly, too stupid, or too weird to be included. Your journal is not supposed to sound smart, although it might if you feel like doing that. Just listen to your inner dialog, connect to your baby and to deeper places inside you. Your journal will eventually become like a personal therapist, after you have been doing it for sometime. In the end you will want to keep a record.

Through writing you can tap into your inner wisdom and answers that are hidden inside your own being. It will also create a precious memory for you and maybe even your family later on after baby is born.

How to start the pregnancy journal?

You can do it using any style you wish but you should keep consistency throughout your pregnancy. You can start each day with recording:

- The date.
- Your weight; weigh yourself every morning when you first get up.
- What you're craving?
- How you're feeling physically and emotionally.
- Dreams you've had.
- Current events that is interesting and noteworthy.
- Thoughts/feelings you've had about the baby.

Creative ways of journaling.

Some entries can be written like a letter to your child. You can start with "My Dear Angel...", "My Little Angel..." "My Dearest Baby..." and write your wishes, express your love and gratitude.

You can also express your feelings and experiences through drawings. You just draw what you feel, what dreams you had and what experiences you had. Often pictures can bypass verbal language and directly reveal inner thoughts and emotions about your pregnancy and baby. You have probably heard the saying 'one picture is worth a thousand words', it is true!

Those of you who like typing and creating something on Internet can start a pregnancy blog - an internet diary; where you write daily entries about your feelings, dreams and wishes. Your pregnancy blog can be private only you can read and access it, or public and other people on Internet can read it also. The beauty of having a blog is that you can add on your photos to your entries, so later on you can see how your body has changed during your pregnancy.

2. **Start daily meditation.** Meditation is a beautiful healthy thing you can do for yourself and your baby during pregnancy. In fact, one of the best ways to intimately connect to your baby is through daily meditation. If you didn't start meditating before pregnancy, start doing it now and enjoy the beautiful time and endless benefits of this simple art.

Here is the simple technique you can do anywhere - at home, at work or outside.

Sit down on a chair or on the floor. Put your hands on your lap, palm side up. Close your eyes and take a deep breath bringing awareness into your body. Feel and envision the space inside you. Feel the body vibrations and energy filling up all your body. Hear its sound, notice the shades, colours and textures within you. For the next several breaths follow the loving sensations inside you. If any thoughts come into your mind, just gently push them away.

Now, place your hands on your belly and imaging your baby inside you. Connect to your baby and send him/her your love and energy through your hands and/or through your heart.

Feel the connecting moment. This meditation will protect your baby and make him/her grow surrounded by your love.

3. **Regular exercise** will make a significant difference in how you feel, increase your energy level, improve your immune system and make you generally healthier and happier.

4. **Self-massage** is great tool for selfcare and nurturing. This self appreciation will also be felt by your baby on a subliminal level. You can do self massage using oils or creams. When massaging the body, it is better to do it with oils. When massaging your face you can do it with a facial cream.

Note: when you start self massage, it is always better to start with massaging your hands first. When that is done you should begin to feel your own energy in your hands and be able to transmit it to other parts of your body.

Here are the steps for facial massage.

1. Massage your hands and fingers for 1-2 minutes. With one of your hands gently squeeze each finger and thumb of the opposite hand. Do it from the base to the top. Then, massage the other hand. Be in the present and really enjoy the feeling of touching your hands. Don't think, just feel. If any other thoughts arrive, gently push them away.

2. Using your index, middle and ring fingers, massage the area above the eyebrows and over the entire forehead using circular motions.

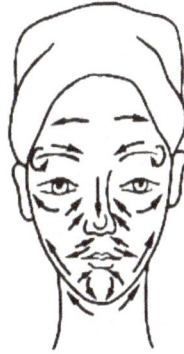

3. Move your fingertips under your eyes and massage very carefully, and then move up and down the sides of your nose. The middle and ring fingers are used and all massage is done in circular movements.
4. Very gently massage the area around your eyes, as well as your temples.
5. Move your fingertips to around your mouth area and massage it.
6. Massage your cheeks moving your fingertips along the lower jaw at first, then along the cheekbones to the middle of your face.
7. Massage the chin and the front of the neck.
8. Spend time rubbing the earlobes. Pull down on the ears gently.
9. Stroke under your chin and throat area using the back of your hand.

5. **Kegel exercises, or pelvic floor exercises,** are the "wonder exercise of pregnancy". These help strengthen the muscles that support the uterus, bladder, and bowels. Strengthening these muscles during pregnancy can help you develop the ability to control your muscles during labour and delivery, also significantly minimize two common problems during pregnancy; bladder control and haemorrhoids. Kegel also helps to strengthen vaginal muscles and increase orgasm.

How to do Kegel Exercises

1) Locate your Kegel muscles first. There a few ways to do this. You can insert a finger into the vagina and try to squeeze the muscles surrounding it. Or you practice stopping the flow of urine when urinating; although you don't want to do this too often during urination because it can actually weaken the muscles, so do it only to feel the pelvic floor muscles.

2) When you have located your Kegel muscles, contract these muscles for 5-10 seconds, then relax, repeating 10-20 times. Make sure to empty your bladder before doing your Kegels!

3) Breathe normally during the exercises, and do this at least three times a day.

4) Try not to move your leg, buttock, or abdominal muscles during the exercises.

You can do it anywhere! Whether you are watching TV, standing in line at the grocery store or are stopped at a red traffic light; fitting Kegels into your busy schedule is easy. Make Kegels a regular part of your fitness routine for life.

Your Weight Gain

Weight gain during pregnancy can differ for most women, but one thing is certain, you should be gaining weight as the months go by. Healthy weight gain during the first trimester is just 450g (1 pound) each month.

Month 2 (5th to 8th Week)

How Is Your Baby?

The second month of pregnancy is one of the most crucial of all months. This is mainly because important changes are taking place in the embryo. It is during this month when your baby's vital organs start to form. Below you will see how your baby's development week by week during the second month.

Week 5: This week your baby resembles a tadpole and is growing very fast. During this week, the heart starts to take shape but it is only a primitive heart which has only two tiny channels called heart tubes. It will also start to beat and will be visible through ultrasound, making it a milestone event.

By the end of the week, many blood vessels will start to form, making up the early parts of the circulatory system. The umbilical which is connected to the placenta is developing: it brings in oxygen, blood and nutrition to your baby. At this stage, your baby is only a few millimetres long and the developing heart is the size a small seed.

Week 6: At this stage, your baby is around 6-6.5 mm (1/8 of an inch). The baby can easily be seen through ultrasound, but has no distinct form as yet. During this week, the vital organs such as the heart, lungs, kidneys and liver will continue to develop. The brain begins to divide into 5 parts and spinal cord (neural tube) which until now has been open, is beginning to close. The facial features, such as baby's jaw, cheeks, and chin, also begin to form. Your baby's heart will beat at least 80 times per minute and will increase as the months go by.

Week 7: By this week, your baby continues to grow rapidly and is now around 0.35 mm to 0.500 mm (⅓ to ½ inches) long, around the same size as a small berry. Facial features are developing and are becoming more and more prominent. The mouth and tongue are forming; the ears are being developed also. Nostrils are becoming more pronounced. The eyes are also quite visible now but no irises (the coloured parts of the eyes). The lower jaw and the vocal cords are becoming more and more distinctive. The digestive tract and kidneys are developing rapidly also.

Week 8: Your baby is now six weeks old from conception. By now a little bit taller than last week and is the same size as a lima bean (around 18 mm long). Eyelids start to grow to cover the eyes. The facial features are becoming more prominent. Elbows, fingers and toes are now growing.

The feet and hand buds have appeared. The baby also starts moving, but may not be felt by its mum till around week 20. The baby's stomach is being created from part of the gut. The teeth begin to develop under the gums. The eyes can now be seen as small hollows on each side of the baby's head. The heart is beating much fast now, around 150 beats per minute.

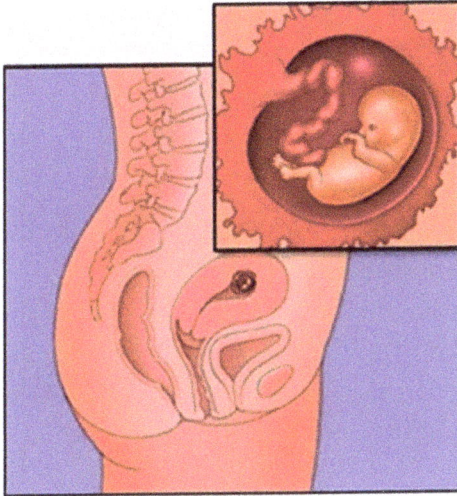

Your baby 2nd month.

Your experiences during the 2nd month of pregnancy.

While you may not be "showing" yet, you can now feel the changes that pregnancy brings to your body. This time, you have already missed a period, which would definitely arouse suspicions that you are pregnant. Other things you might be feeling:

- Nausea or morning sickness, although it can occur any time of the day.
- Breast tenderness and darkening of the nipples.
- Selective reactions to certain foods.
- Recurrent head aches or feelings of dizziness.

- Constipation and/or bloating.
- Clothes start to feel tight, especially around the waist.
- Emotional changes: irritability, unstable moods, tearfulness, anxiety.
- Changes in your face: face isn't looking the same as it was pre-pregnancy.
- Visible veins on the chest and abdomen, blood vessels expand to meet the needs of the growing foetus.
- "Spider veins" on the thighs look like thin purplish-red lines. They usually disappear after delivery.
- Fatigue and tiredness.
- Excessive salivation.
- White colour vaginal discharge.

Bleeding, Pain and Other Problems

Vaginal bleeding is a worry at any stage of pregnancy, but it is fairly common during the first trimester. During this month, there are a number of reasons why this happens. Bleeding may be caused by implantation, or can occur after sexual intercourse as the cervix is more prone to contact. Bleeding caused after sexual intercourse or caused by implantation should be light to medium only. In cases of severe bleeding, contact your medical professional right away.

Dizziness is a common symptom during the second month. However, if you are experiencing severe dizziness which comes with the vaginal bleeding and abdominal pain, seek medical help immediately. These symptoms may indicate an ectopic pregnancy, which has a life threatening complication.

Your weight.

You may notice yourself gaining a few kilos. Or, if you are experiencing morning sickness, you may also lose a bit of weight. Healthy weight gain during the first trimester should only be

500g (1 pound) each month. Gaining lots of weight throughout your pregnancy can be very bad for your health or that of your baby's. Your doctor should take note of these changes and make some dietary suggestions if necessary.

Physical symptoms.

Many of the physical symptoms that you may have during this month are not new ones. You more than likely have had similar ones already in the first month. Or you may be like many other women who have not had any problem at all.

Morning Sickness.

To avoid the scourges of morning sickness, it is important for you to change your eating habits. Choose foods that are easy to digest and low in fat.

Eat lots of small meals throughout the day to prevent your stomach from becoming completely empty. Frequent snacking on crackers, dry biscuits and wheat bread can help to combat the nausea. If you feel tired, take a break from what you are doing and get some rest. Get as much protein and iron as you can, since these will help combat fatigue also. Keep yourself hydrated, especially if you are throwing up due to morning sickness; try to drink lots of water.

Acupressure, acupuncture, relaxation and herbal remedies can be very useful for morning sickness relief also. But it is a good idea to check with a professional if the herbs are safe.

Dizziness.

Dizziness is caused by a drop in your blood pressure or sugar level. To avoid the occasional dizzy spells, try not to stand for long periods of time. Get up slowly from a bed or from a chair. Make sure that you stop what you are doing and just sit or lie down when you feel faint, you don't want to fall over.

Breast tenderness.

Your breasts may begin to feel tender and sore, so invest in good bra one with good support. A supportive bra can make things more comfortable as you go about with your day.

Healthy things to do during the 2nd month.

You should continue doing regular exercises, since moving around makes you fit and makes it easier for you to adapt to the changes in your body. The best exercises you can do are yoga, stretching, walking and swimming. In fact, you can simply move around the house and do some chores to keep yourself active, if you can't get out and about.

You should continue all the healthy things we discussed in the first month of your pregnancy:

- writing in your "Pregnancy Diary".
- daily meditation.
- regular exercise and/or yoga.
- facial self-massage.

Don't forget to practice Kegel exercises throughout the pregnancy as these are very important for your health and wellbeing. Also simply keep doing them even after pregnancy for health.

What can you do new his month to make yourself feel better?

Self-massage of the scalp.

Scalp self-massage will help you to relieve stress, cope with headaches, make you sleep better and rejuvenate you during the day. When you do self-massage turn on some pleasant relaxing music. But you can choose to do it in silence. Whatever feels better for you, just do it. Let's start the scalp massage now.

1. Massage your hands for 1-2 minutes to feel the energy in your own hands.

2. Place your hands on the sides of your face: palms on cheeks and fingertips right behind your ears. With circular movements (clockwise) massage the area behind your ears from the top to the bottom of your hair line.

3. Spread out your fingers and with your fingertips make stroking movements from the top of forehead to the top of the head. Then do the same stroking movements on the sides of your head.

4. With your fingers still spread out, massage your scalp making big circles (clockwise) around 5-7 cm in diameter. Start from the sides of the head moving to the top of the head, than towards the forehead and down towards the neck.

5. Continue to massage with small circular movements (clockwise) from the sides to the top of the head and down to the neck.

6. Take long deep breaths while massaging your scalp. Focus just on the sensations of touching. If any thoughts come gently push them away.

7. Repeat the massage movements from the beginning but change the direction of the gentle circles to counter-clockwise.

Allocate time for self-massage from 5-20 min a day, but you can do it as often as you need to relax.

Listening to music.

Music has a powerful effect on our emotions. A quiet, gentle lullaby can calm us down and a majestic chorus can make us swell with excitement. Also, music can affect the way we think. It doesn't exactly mean that music makes us smarter but music seems to prime our brains for certain kinds of thinking. After listening to classical music, adults can concentrate better and solve mathematical problems faster than people who didn't listen to such music. Classical music seems to have a priming effect on our ability to concentrate. Many experts believe that children exposed to classical music in the womb are more apt to having positive physical and mental development after birth. If you follow the expert's advice, then choose Mozart, Bach, Vivaldi and Chopin.

Music made for Meditation is also very beneficial: it promotes healing and is able to create a calming effect, helping a person to relax the parts of the mind that constantly chatter and interrupt.

> *Advice: make some time and listen to relaxing, calming and soothing music. During pregnancy, classical and meditation music is probably the best choice to listen to. Try not to listen to heavy metal or heavy rock as this has been proven to cause bad vibrations, in animals and even plants.*

Month 3rd (9th to 12th Week)

This is the last month of the first trimester. The baby is developing rapidly and his/her basic physiology will be fully developed during this month. If morning sickness has been a disturbance, you may finally get some relief. Even urinary urges and severe fatigue will become less troubling or may even disappear at the end of this month.

> **Week 9:** Your baby is about 2.3 cm now and weighs less than 2 grams. The baby's essential body parts and organs have now developed and are all formed, although they will go through a lot of fine tuning over the next few months to come. The organs, muscles and nerves are already functioning. It is still too soon to tell the baby's gender since the external sex organs are not distinguishable yet for the next few weeks.
>
> The baby's eyes are fully formed but are still covered by eyelids, which will open by around the 27th week. The

placenta is already developed enough and is already producing hormones for your baby.

Week 10: Your baby is about 3-4 cm long and weighs about 3.5 grams. Most of the vital organs liver, kidneys, intestines, brain, and lungs are in place and already started to function. The stomach already is producing digestive juices and the kidneys are already starting to filter and produce urine. If your baby is a boy, his internal sex organs will already begin to produce testosterone.

The baby's fingers and toes are no longer joined by webbing, and tiny nails are already forming on each of the digits. Hair is also starting to grow on the skin. Aside from these developments, your baby can already bend its limbs and flex the wrists. The spine is clearly visible underneath translucent skin.

Week 11: Your baby is already 5 cm long and weighs about 9 grams. The hands can now open and close, forming firsts. Bones are already hardening and Baby is already busy stretching and kicking, but you still won't notice the movement for the next month or two.

Hair follicles are starting to form: fingernails and toenails are starting to grow. You still can't tell the baby's sex yet but if it's a girl the ovaries are developing at this time. What you also can see clearly at this stage is your baby has distinct human looking traits with their limbs in front of the body, distinctive ears, open nasal passages, a tongue and a palate in the mouth and visible nipples.

Week 12: Your baby starts to make some dramatic advances and soon will develop reflexes. The baby's weight is now about 15 grams and approximately 6 cm long from crown to bottom. Good news at this point is the chance of miscarriage drops considerably after this week because the most critical developments are complete. The digestive system is beginning to practice contractive movements, so your baby is starting to digest food, the bone marrow is producing white blood cells, part of baby's immune system which protects it from infections. The pituitary glands also have started making hormones for growth. The fingers can now open and close, the mouth can make sucking movements and eye muscles begin to contract. The baby now starts to respond to stimuli and will move when you press on your abdomen, although you won't be able to feel the baby move yet. The intestine is beginning to work and the kidneys are excreting urine into the bladder. The nerve cells are now multiplying rapidly, forming synapses in the brain.

At this time period the baby's face already looks very human, with the eyes, ears and nose already in place.

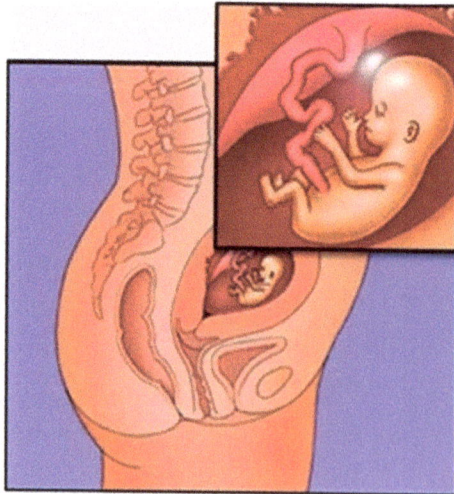

Your baby at the 3rd month.

Your experiences during the 3rd month of pregnancy.

Your uterus now continues to expand, and you may notice that your waistline has started to thickened a bit. By the twelfth week, your uterus has now expanded to the size of a grapefruit. While you may still not be "showing," you may feel uncomfortable wearing your tight clothes and may prefer to wear looser ones instead.

You may continue to experience most of the symptoms from the first and second month, such as:

- Nausea and 'morning sickness'.
- Dizziness and occasional faintness.
- Fatigue and tiredness.
- Mood swings: from elation and joy to sudden tearfulness and anxiety.
- Indigestion problems such as bloating, heartburn, constipation
- Food aversion and cravings
- Headaches
- Breast changes: heaviness, tenderness, darkened areolas and goose bumps on them, visible veins and enlarged nipples.

The good news is that by the end of the third month, you should begin to feel more energetic if you've been experiencing fatigue. Morning sickness should begin to lessen and you may start to notice an increase in appetite.

Your oil glands also become more active. The excess oil tends to make hair and skin shinier, but for many women it may also mean acne outbreaks.

Note: *You may be feeling perfectly well; you may be experiencing only a few minor symptoms or may be you got all symptoms right from the start. Always remember that every pregnancy is different and the experiences are different.*

Varicose veins.

Some women may notice varicose veins which can happen in those who are predisposed to the condition. Varicose veins usually show up on your legs, just under the skin's surface, but you can get them in other parts of your body too.

Symptoms of this condition are visible swollen veins, pain in the veins and feelings of heaviness in the legs.

What to do to prevent varicose veins from progressing?

- Avoid excessive weight gain.
- Do not stand for a long time.
- When sitting, if possible raise your legs above hip level.
- When sleeping or lying down put a pillow under your feet to keep them a bit higher than your normal sleeping position. This improves blood flow and stops blood congestion in the legs.
- Do not sit cross legged for a long time.
- Avoid heavy lifting.
- Wear special stockings that support the leg muscles.
- Do not wear tight fitting clothes, socks with elastic in the upper part.
- Wear soft comfortable shoes.
- Do not smoke.
- Do light physical exercises, such as daily deal brisk walking for 20-30 minutes.
- Take plenty of vitamin "C" which makes your veins stronger.

Surgical treatment of varicose veins during pregnancy is not recommended. It can be done after birth if the condition does not improve. Often varicose veins get better after birth.

When to Contact Your Doctor?

You should be visiting your doctor around every 4 weeks for the first and second trimester. Your doctor will continue to track your progress and note changes in your body, any weight gain and the growth of your baby.

Most pregnancy symptoms will probably feel a little uncomfortable, so be sure to pay attention if they start to become severe. Seek medical care immediately if you experience any heavy bleeding, bad stomach pain and severe constipation, or if you are vomiting uncontrollably.

Your Weight Gain

Like the first and second month of pregnancy, a healthy weight gain should be around 500g for the whole month. Your doctor will continue to take note of these changes and will give you recommendations for any weight issues if there are any.

Sex during the First Trimester (1st to 3rd Month)

Many women ask this question: is it safe to have sex during pregnancy? The answer is yes. In fact, many women continue to do so even until their last month. You will not injure your baby by making love. The uterus, thick mucus plug in the cervix and amniotic fluid protects the baby.

While sex is quite safe, in the first three months of pregnancy you may find that your uncomfortable symptoms may lower your sex drive. Many women feel too tired or nauseous to have sex. Breast tenderness, bloating, and the increased need to urinate can take a toll on your sex drive. Not all women experience the same things, so listen to what your body is telling you and do what feels comfortable.

The best sexual positions during first trimester are:

- Woman on top. This is a great position during pregnancy as you're in control of the depth of penetration, the speed you can go with, as fast or slow as you like and the movement.

- Sideways. This position has you and your partner lying on their sides facing one another.
- Spooning. This position requires you and your partner to lie on your sides, with your partner facing your back.
- From behind. "Doggy style' allows for deeper penetration and is often very pleasurable for both parties.
- Sitting.

Healthy things to do during the 3rd month.

You should continue all the healthy things you have already been doing such as journaling, meditation, self-massage and listening to music. These are all great to do! But this month you may be interested to learn about how you can communicate with your body. Did you know your body talks? But first you need to listen and second you need to ask for the answer.

Talking to your body during pregnancy.

Yes, you can talk to your body! You can talk to your organs, you limbs, your head, your uterus and your child!

Talking to your body is a well-known technique from ancient times. Shamans and witch-doctors used this technique to heal people from different ailments. Even though some people may consider it weird, the technique works very well if you know how to practice it.

Complete relaxation is the key to successful body talk. Generally, people who meditate regularly find it easier to communicate with their bodies than people who don't meditate. The reason for this is meditation makes you become more in tune with your body so the 'body talk' becomes easy to understand.

Now, how to do 'body talk'?

1. Completely accept the notion that our bodies are not just bio-physical machines but spiritual beings. The common spirit (or energy) runs through us all.

2. Before you start the 'body talk" you need to relax as much as you can. Meditate, listen to music and/or do yoga; whichever makes you feel completely relaxed.

3. In a relaxed state, focus on the part of the body (or organ) that you want to heal or talk to. If this is your heart, then focus on your heart. You can put your hand on the area of your heart to help you to focus. Visualise it. Start your talk with: "My dear heart, I am so grateful for the work you do. You have helped me during all my life. Thank you so much. Please help me to go through my pregnancy and carry a healthy child."

Add on whatever you feel like saying, whatever your problems are and whatever you need to say.

If you want to talk to your feet, then focus on your feet. You can pat your feet, touch them or just mentally focus on them and say: "My dear feet. I love you so much. You carry my body from the time of my first step. Please help me to carry my pregnancy. Please be good, be light and healthy…" Visualise blood flowing up and down gracefully to your feet without any stasis or blockages.

If you need to be healed from a cold or from any other infections; you can visualize your white blood cells fighting against viruses or bacteria like soldiers fighting their enemies. You can ask them to fight better and to make you free from the infection.

There is no limit to this. You can talk to any part of the body, organ or system which needs healing. You can talk as long as you wish, there is no limit. The most important things are the relaxation and the focusing.

The more you do it, the easier it becomes. Learning a bit of basic anatomy will help with visualisation also. The more clearly you visualise inside your body, the more healing power your talk has. For example, you want to talk to your heart, look up basic heart anatomy (4 heart chambers and the blood flow).

If you want to talk to your baby, look up the anatomy of your pregnant uterus during this time of pregnancy. What is the size of your baby, what organs are developed, what senses are developed at this time?

Knowing the anatomy of your body brings you a certain healing power!

Month 4 (13th to 16th Week)

Congratulations, you have now reached the second trimester of your pregnancy. Three months have already gone by and you now only have to wait for six more months before you finally see your little bundle of joy. Most of the uncomfortable symptoms during the first trimester such as vomiting, nausea and morning sickness will start to lessen and eventually stop during this month. During the coming months, you will experience some new changes in your body as your baby continues to grow.

> **Week 13:** Your baby is 11 weeks into development and is growing quite quickly. The Baby now measures about 8 cm (3 inches) from top of the head to the bottom and weighs about 23 grams. Your baby's weight gain has been quite rapid, considering that he started out at only 2 grams the month before. The eyes are already in the correct position. The ankles and wrists are forming, and toes and fingers are already separate from each other. The baby's head is still quite big in proportion to his body, but the features are almost all correct. The intestines are slowly shifting into position away from the umbilical cord and into the baby's abdomen. External genitalia are becoming more and more pronounced now. The child can open and close his mouth and can now also place his thumb inside the mouth and suckle it. The baby's movement is a lot more now and your

baby can move its legs and arms around easily. The placenta covering baby is now fully formed, and the umbilical cord continues to thicken, carrying more and more nourishment.

Week 14: The baby now measures somewhere around 9 to 10 cm and weighs about 40 grams. The facial features are developed. The ears have moved and are now located on the sides of the head. The eyes are gradually moving towards the front of the face. The neck starts to elongate and the chin is more and more prominent. *Lanugo* or fine, short hairs are starting to cover the entire body. This hair growth is quite helpful in keeping the baby warm, since there is not much body fat yet. The baby begins to respond to outside influences and may move away when your abdomen is poked. The vocal cords, windpipes, larynx and gullet have all developed more. The kidneys are producing urine and the ovaries (in girls) are moving down towards the pelvis. In boys, the prostate gland is developing. The baby's mouth is continuously moving, making sucking motions, opening and closing and smiling. These movements help give his facial muscles a workout, which helps develop the shape and size of its little cheeks. Your baby looks more and more human now. The eyes, ears, lips are now in place. The jaw has properly formed and the palate is now closing up. The placenta is fully developed and functional, but it is still larger than your baby.

Week 15: The baby now weighs 60 to 70 grams and is about 10-11 cm long. The baby is now fully covered with lanugo, and hair is starting to sprout on top of the head as well. Lanugo usually disappears right before birth, but some babies still come out quite hairy and furry. His skin is still quite thin, making blood vessels clearly visible through it.

The baby can make breathing movements with his nose and mouth in preparation for life outside of the womb. The baby can already hiccup, but can't make any sound yet as it is still immersed in fluid. Aside from these developments, the baby can also move his fingers and toes and do some fine dancing motions. It is still too early to feel these movements and as you need to wait until about 18th-20th week before you start feeling them. Your baby's organs are now increasing in size, especially the circulatory system and heart. It continues to pump 11 litres of blood every day. The baby continues to make breathing actions, inhaling and exhaling amniotic fluid to prepare its air sacs for real breathing. The bones are starting to get harder, and will continue on for the rest of the time. This process is called "ossification." The liver starts to secrete bile that is essential for fat digestion. The pancreas also starts to produce insulin that converts sugar into energy.

Week 16: You are now at the end of your fourth month, "congratulations" and your baby continues to grow more and more as the weeks tick by. Your baby now measures nearly 12 cm from head to bottom and weighs around 100 grams. The ears are now in place; this means that baby can already hear you and other voices from the outside fairly well. The baby continues to make jerky movements with his hands and feet, and you may start feeling some movements now. Although many mums still don't feel anything, but don't worry about it, if you do not feel any movement you will soon. The baby's tiny muscles are getting stronger, allowing baby to stretch the body. The facial muscles are gaining strength and facial expressions are becoming more regular. The ears are already moving close to their final position. The eyes, although still closed, are already working. They can already notice changes in light and move from side to side. At this point the toenails have also started to grow.

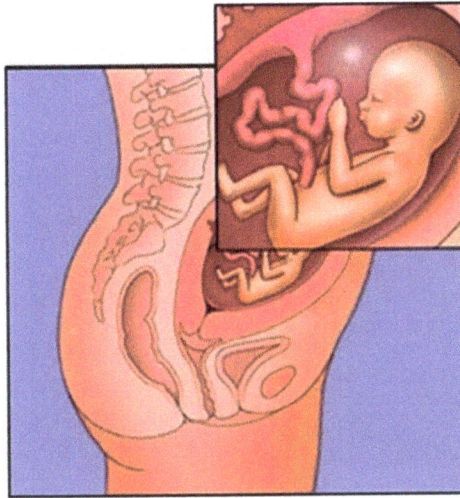

Your baby at 4th month.

Your experiences during the 4th month.

You are starting to show more now as your uterus is expanding. Your breasts are growing and your blood volume has increased causing you to gain weight. You will now find that a lot of the uncomfortable symptoms that you had during the first trimester are gone. Although you now are faced with a whole new set of symptoms.

Here are some new symptoms that you may experience this month:

- **Insomnia.** You may start having difficulties in sleeping as you get bigger. More than 70% of all women experience insomnia during their second and third trimesters of pregnancy. There are many probable causes of sleep difficulties that include more discomfort, a more frequent need to urinate, leg cramps can start and other pregnancy annoyances.
- **Gas.** Gas is also a common symptom during pregnancy because your body is producing high levels of progesterone.

This hormone relaxes the muscles in your digestive tract leading to flatulence, gas and bloating.

- **Nasal Congestion.** This symptom is common during pregnancy and is caused by swelling of the mucous membranes in the nose. This doesn't mean you have a cold, it is just one of the new annoyances that will come and go during the next six months.
- **Salivation.** Hormonal changes also play a role in causing this symptom. Your body may also be producing more saliva to help relieve heartburn, since it neutralizes gastric acid.
- **Skin Changes.** You may also begin to experience skin changes. The increase in your blood circulation makes your cheeks rosier and causes your face to appear brighter. The oil glands are also working overtime making your face shiny. These changes can result in what is called a "pregnancy glow," but too much oil can also cause acne outbreaks. Some women may also get a blotchy skin tone.
- **Haemorrhoids.** Haemorrhoids are caused by pressure placed on the rectal veins. They typically appear during the second trimester, but not all women get them.
- **Shortness of Breath.** You may feel like you are always out of breath, and this is because your uterus is slowly pressing up against the lungs.
- **Bleeding Gums and Nose.** The high blood volume in your system increases the possibility of bleeding from gums and from your nose. While these symptoms are not of a serious nature, regular nosebleeds can be quite annoying, especially if you have to go to work or out of the house a lot.
- **Achy Feet.** Your increasing weight may put pressure on your knees and feet, making your legs feel heavier and your feet sore, especially towards the end of the day.

Although you have developed these new symptoms, some women will still have the old pregnancy symptoms from the months before. These include:

- Frequent urination
- Nausea and vomiting
- Vaginal discharge
- Constipation
- Heartburn
- Light headedness and feelings of dizziness
- Tender or swollen breasts
- Shift in emotions and anxiety
- Fatigue

Healthy things to do during the 4th month.

There are many things you can do to be more comfortable during this month. If you have made some dietary changes during the last weeks, continue following on with the diet. If you have not changed your diet, then now is perfect time to do it. Make sure you eat whole grains, vegetables, low fat foods and dairy products. A good diet can improve your bowel movement, relieve any constipation issues and ease haemorrhoids problems.

Continue to do regular exercises, these don't have to be strenuous just as long as you are doing something. A quick 20-30 minute walk can make a big difference. Meditation, prenatal yoga and Kegel exercises will help to keep you strong and prepare your body for labour.

Another common symptom you may get is insomnia; this can be caused by a wide range of factors. Most of the time any sleeping difficulties you have, could stem from other pregnancy discomforts. To stay comfortable at night, invest in a supportive pillow and sleep on your side, try not to sleep on your back anymore. You can reduce leg cramps and fatigue by having a relaxing bath, a warm shower or a soothing massage, or a self-massage like we covered earlier. You can also make use of a humidifier or saline solution to help keep your nose from feeling stuffy.

Use oil-free or organic products on your skin. Organic skin care products are safe for you and your baby, but can help in keeping your skin free from shine and acne.

Have you mastered the 'body talk' which we discussed last month? Hopefully it is helping you to cope with the problems and complaints of pregnancy. Now we will introduce another useful tool to make you feel better. This tool is positive affirmations.

Positive Affirmations during Pregnancy.

Believe it or not, but positive affirmations are a great help during pregnancy. If you don't program your own mind, then something else or someone else will. And this something or someone may not program your mind the way you want. They may program it in an opposite way. Negative comments, negative information and negative energy can program your mind and affect your health, even your pregnancy negatively.

To take full control of your own mind and your own life as well, start doing positive affirmations now.

Just to remind you: positive affirmations are positive statements that are used to change your daily thoughts and eventually they can change your mindset, feelings and even life. You can write your own affirmations and repeat them whenever you like. Remember they should be in the present tense, as if what you wish to happen is already happening.

For example, a friend of mine who suddenly fell pregnant at 41 with her first child, would say, "I am a healthy woman and my baby is a healthy child." She said this every morning, even during the difficult times when she experienced severe morning sickness and had a period when doctors thought she may lose her baby. She says she remembers visualizing her healthy baby in her arms when she did her affirmations. She feels it really helped her from falling into despair. Fortunately, her pregnancy eventuated with giving birth to a healthy boy. She says she visualised this moment when she was doing her positive affirmations.

If you choose to write your own affirmations, start with phrases like:

- I am (healthy, grateful, lucky .....)
- My body is (strong, healthy, and beautiful.....)
- My baby is (strong, healthy, and beautiful...)
- My pregnancy is (healthy, natural, easy...)
- My body knows how to cope with pregnancy.
- I love my pregnancy.

Women use positive affirmations for many reasons: to overcome fear, to feel confident, to remind them that pregnancy is not an illness, to feel stronger, more loved and loving. While affirmations are simple and easy, they are also effective for many women.

Here are more samples:

- I know how to take care of myself in pregnancy.
- My body knows how to give birth.
- Birth is safe for me and my baby.
- My baby will be born at the perfect time.
- I am connected to my baby.
- My baby will find the perfect position for birth.
- I love my pregnancy and my baby.
- My baby loves me.
- I am a strong woman.
- Contractions help to bring my baby.
- I will make the right decisions for my baby.

- My pregnant body is beautiful.
- My baby knows I love him.
- I accept the help of others.
- I accept my labour and birth.
- I am surrounded by those who love and respect me.
- I trust my body.
- I know how to take care of my baby.
- My baby feels my love.
- I will make plenty of breast milk for my baby.

You can write your affirmations in a diary or write them on your laptop, or notepad. Some women use index cards. Consider using your affirmations as a part of your relaxation routine during or after meditation/yoga. They also make really nice mantras for labour! Certainly, you can chant them!

Your Weight Gain

Normal weight gain during the second trimester is 500 grams a week, which means that by the end of this month, you should have gained another 2 kilos.

Month 5 (17th to 20th Week)

By the time you get to the end off this period you will be midway through your pregnancy. One of the most exciting things about being pregnant will happen this month. You will start to feel the baby move. Ultrasounds become more interesting to watch as your baby's hands and legs are fully visible and almost perfectly shaped. Overall, this is a good month and can be one of the most rewarding in the of your whole pregnancy.

> **Week 17:** On the 17th week of pregnancy, foetal age of 15 weeks your baby's length is about 13 to 14 cm (5.5 inches) top of head to bottom and it would be about

23 cm (9 inches) if the baby could lay flat. The baby now weighs about 150 g.

Body fat on the baby is now starting to form, but the child is still quite lean and the skin is still quite translucent. The growth of fat will give the baby energy and help keep your baby warm after being born. The baby's eyes are looking forward now, but they are still shut tight. The retina has become sensitive to light. The baby's first stool, meconium, composed of products of cell loss, digestive secretion and swallowed amniotic fluid, is accumulating in the bowel track. The rubbery cartilage that will become the skeleton is starting to harden into bone.

Week 18: This week the foetus measures about 15 cm and weighs almost 200 grams. Baby can now hear sounds: hear your heart beating, your breathing, your stomach rumbling or blood moving through the umbilical cord. Try to make sure your body noises are calm, relaxed and not disturbed by stress! At this time even a loud noise may startled the baby. The skin is building a protective wax layer called vernix, which is a white cheese like material on the skin. The lungs continue to form preparing the baby for its first breath after birth. Vocal chords are ready to function but without air don't make a sound yet. The baby can cry, yawn, hiccup, sleep and have awakening pattern similar to a newborn. The baby has its own favourite positions for sleep and rest.

Week 19: At 19 weeks, the foetus lengths is around 17 cm (6.5 inches) and weights about 250 gram. In girls, the organs like vagina, uterus, and fallopian tubes are formed and in place. In boys, the genitals are distinct and recognizable.

Interesting point: If it is a girl she has about 6 million eggs in her ovaries but this amount will lessen and by birth she will have around 1-2 million eggs in her ovaries. By the time her menstruation begins, only about 400,000 ovarian eggs are left to develop into mature eggs.

The baby's muscles and bones are growing rapidly and some women start to feel strong kicks inside now.

Week 20: You made it. Congratulations! Now you are half-way through your pregnancy at the 20 weeks mark; the mid-point. The baby is about 17 cm long from head to bottom and about 25.5 cm from head to heels, and weighs about 310 grams. The baby can hear and recognize its mother's voice. Start saying nice words to your little one and show him/her your love. Talking to your belly, singing songs, telling kind loving stories, all these will benefit to the baby's development and forming its personality. Familiar voices, music, and sounds that baby becomes accustomed to while in the womb often have a calming effect after birth.

Your baby's personality is now starting to form very intensely right now! Don't miss this wonderful opportunity to teach your little one something nice, loving and kind.

Your baby's movements become very obvious and with a stethoscope you can hear their heart beating. The toenails and fingernails are growing and the skin is getting thicker.

Note: Body measurement of the length of the baby.

Before 20 weeks babies are measured from the top of the head to the bottom. After 20 weeks, they are measured from head to heel. This is because a baby's legs are curled up against the body during the first half of pregnancy and very hard to measure.

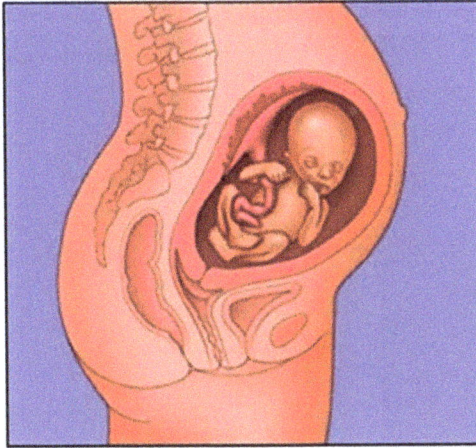

Your baby at 5th month of pregnancy.

Your experiences during the 5th month of pregnancy.

Everybody is different and every pregnancy is also different. You may experience all the symptoms described here, or may experience just a few or none at all. You may also have other less common symptoms, this is quite OK. But here is what many pregnant women feel during this month:

- *More energy.* Many women have more energy this month as the disturbing symptoms of the 1st trimester are gone and the difficulties of the late months have not come yet.
- *Increased appetite.* The cause of increased appetite during this month is the growing baby which needs certain vitamins and nutrients; and also the end of the morning sickness.
- *Baby's movements have become obvious.* Around the 20th week you should start feeling your baby moves inside you.
- *Pains and aches from the pressure and stretched ligaments* (back pains, low abdomen and sides of the body aches, and leg and feet aches).

- *Leg cramps.* This happens for number of reasons. First, your muscles are bearing more weight nowadays. Second, you may have a shortage of nutrients and salts, such as calcium or magnesium, circulating in your blood (due to high demand for these nutrients when you're pregnant).
- *Forgetfulness.* The findings why pregnancy can affect your memory are inconsistent. It is probably all related to hormonal changes but not all women complain about it. Many pregnant women can function mentally as well as normal, when they are not pregnant.
- *Heartburn, indigestion, flatulence and bloating.* All these symptoms happen due to baby's pressure on your stomach, intestines and bowel. Hormonal changes also contribute to these problems.
- *Nasal congestion, nose bleed, ear stiffness.* Nasal and ear congestion during pregnancy occurs when high levels of oestrogens and progesterone increase blood flow to all the body's mucous membranes, including the nose, which causes them to swell and soften and often leads to nosebleeds during pregnancy as well.
- *Gums bleed.* Your gums bleed when you floss or brush because your higher progesterone levels make your gums more sensitive to the bacteria in plaque.
- *Mild swelling on the ankles and feet and occasionally hands and face.* As your baby grows, your uterus puts pressure on blood vessels in your pelvis. This particularly affects the large veins that receive blood from your limbs. Pressure from this trapped blood forces water down and out through tiny vessels (capillaries) into the tissues of your feet and ankles.

- *Varicose veins and haemorrhoids.* Pregnancy makes you more prone to haemorrhoids, as well as to varicose veinsfor a variety of reasons. Your growing uterus puts pressure on the pelvic veins and the inferior vena cava, a large vein on the right side of the body that receives blood from the lower limbs. This can slow the return of blood from the lower half of your body, which increases the pressure on the veins below your uterus and causes them to become more dilated or swollen. In addition, an increase in the hormone progesterone during pregnancy causes the walls of your veins to relax, allowing them to swell more easily.
- *Skin colour changes on the abdomen and face.* These changes are triggered by hormonal changes during pregnancy, which stimulate a temporary increase in your body's production of melanin, the natural substance that gives colour to hair, skin, and eyes.
- *Constipation.* Increase of hormone progesterone contributes to constipation by slowing down your intestinal tract. Haemorrhoids can also make constipated.
- *Vaginal discharge.* The cause of it is an increased oestrogen production and greater blood flow to the vagina. This discharge is made up of secretions from the cervix and vagina, old cells from the walls of the vagina, and normal bacterial flora from the vagina.
- *Feeling hot when everybody else is cool.* During pregnancy your hormonal level is high and that increases the blood flow to the skin making you feel hot.
- *Dizziness.* High level of progesterone causes your blood vessels to relax and widen, increasing the blood flow to your baby but slowing the return of blood to your brain. You can also feel dizzy when your blood sugar level is low.

Healthy things to do during the 5th month of pregnancy.

Since your appetite has improved, you have to make sure that you eat healthy food now. Also remember that you are eating for two, this means eating nutritious food and not just doubling the amount of food you are eating as this can be dangerous. Fresh fruits and vegies, whole grain, low fat dairy products, lean meat and chicken, fish and seafood are the best choices at this time.

Try to manage your pains and aches using alternative methods without taking any drugs (read the chapter "Pain management during pregnancy").

Cramping:

When you get a leg cramp, straighten your leg from the heel, gently flexing your "toes towards your nose". This can be uncomfortable but will ease the spasm and help the pain to go dissipate. To prevent cramps, take multivitamins with calcium and magnesium and do calf stretches. To do calf stretches, stand a metre from a wall and lean forwards with your arms outstretched to touch the wall. Keep the soles of your feet flat on the floor. Hold for five seconds. Repeat the exercise for five minutes, three times a day, especially before going to bed.

Forgetfulness:

The best way to deal with forgetfulness and absentmindedness is to do regular meditation. Meditation will improve your memory, make your mind clearer and you become more attentive.

Heartburn:

To relieve heartburn avoid food and beverages that can aggravate the condition like, carbonated drinks; alcohol, which you should avoid during pregnancy anyway; caffeine; chocolate; acidic foods like citrus fruits and juices, tomatoes, mustard, and vinegar; processed meats; or spicy highly seasoned foods, fried, and fatty foods. Eat several small meals throughout the day. Try chewing gum after eating. Chewing gum stimulates your salivary glands, and saliva can help neutralize acid. Sleep propped up with several pillows or a wedge. Elevating your upper body will help keep your stomach acids down and will aid your digestion. Bend at the knees instead of at the waist. If natural methods do not help, ask your doctor about prescribing an antacid. Be careful about antacids which contains sodium bicarbonate (baking soda) as they can increase water retention in your body.

Swelling:

To reduce swelling of your feet and ankles try to put your feet up whenever possible especially at night. Don't cross your legs or ankles while sitting. Stretch your legs frequently. Stretch your legs out, heel first, and gently flex your foot to stretch your calf muscles. Rotate your ankles and wiggle your toes. Take regular breaks from sitting or standing. Do more walking and exercise regularly, don't become stationary.

Special exercises to improve blood circulation and strengthen the body.

This set of exercises involves many important groups of muscles: abdominal muscles, legs, thighs, pelvis, calf muscles, arms and shoulders, back and neck muscles. The purpose of these exercises is to stretch and strengthen the muscles and prevent your body from becoming floppy and weak, prepare yourself for labour and make the recovery process after labour faster.

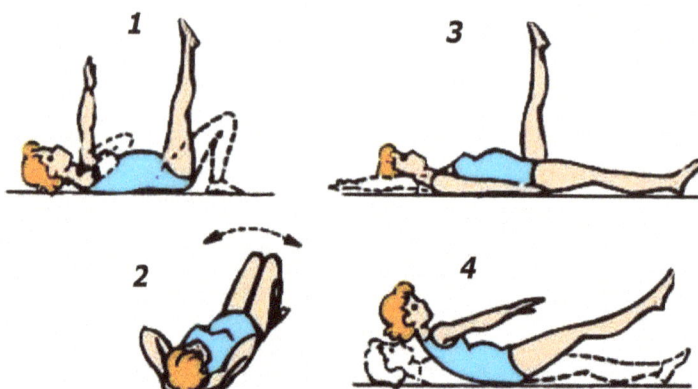

1. Lie down on your back; flex your knees. Put your hands on the shoulders. Simultaneously, lift one leg and both arms up then put them down. Then, lift another leg and both arms up and put them down. Repeat 10 times (see figure 1 above).

2. Lie down on your back; flex your knees. Lock your fingers together and put them behind your head. Keep your knees together then turn to the right and then the left side stretching the hip and thigh muscles, repeat 10 times (see figure 2).

3. Lie down on your back, legs straightened and your arms placed flat along your sides. Simultaneously lift one leg straight up to 90 degrees, at the same time move the opposite arm over your head and lay flat on the floor above your head. Then, put the leg down and your arms go back along the sides of your body. Do the same movements with another leg repeat 10 times (see figure 3).

4. Lie down on your back; legs straightened and your arms are along your sides. Lift your right leg up 45 degrees above the floor while lifting your body off the floor and raising your arms up also. Then lower yourself slowly go

down and lift again with the opposite leg repeat 10 times (see figure 4).

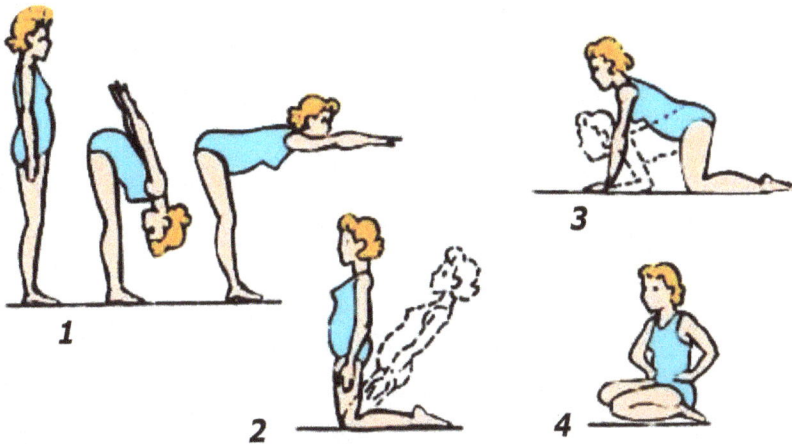

1. Stand up straight; your arms are down by your sides. Bend forward and down keeping your knees straight, your arms should be flat along your back pointing up. Now, move your arms forward keeping your body and arms straight. Make an angle between your body and legs of 90 degrees. Stay in this position for a few seconds and stand up straight again, putting your arms down along your sides. Repeat 10 times (Figure 1).

2. Raise yourself to your knees, your arms down along your sides. Swing your body backwards trying to keep balance and bring it back straight again. Repeat 5 times (Figure 2)

3. With your knees and forearm on the floor straighten your arms with a push up motion, repeat 10 times (figure 3).

4. Sit on your feet with your hands on the waist line. Twist your body left and then right as much as you can, repeat 10 times (figure 4).

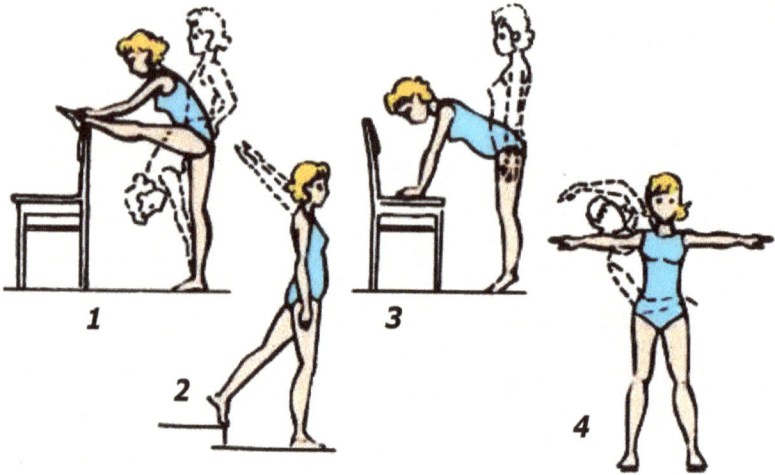

1. Get a stabile chair one that firm on the floor and will not move. Or you can use the back of a lounge chair or desk, as long as it will not tilt or move. Put one leg on the back of the chair. Now move you fingers down towards your toes. Stand up again then bend your body forward towards the foot which is on the back of the chair. Then change legs and continue the same actions on this side repeat 10 times on each leg (figure 1).

   Note: do this exercise only if you are fit enough to do it. Make sure to use only safe equipment that will not fall on you while you're exercising.

2. Stand on one step; use only a bottom step with a good flat floor. Your arms are down along your sides. Step down with one foot and lift your arms above your head at the same time. Step back up and put your hands down. Do the same with the other leg, repeat 10 times (figure 2).

3. Get a safe chair and put your hands on the seat firmly. Your feet are on the floor. Move your heels up and down

10 times keeping your toes on the floor. Then stand up straight and move your heels up and down 10 times keeping the toes on the floor (figure 3).

4. Stand up straight; put your feet apart and your arms out the sides. Bend your body left with the left arms goes down in front of the belly and the right arm goes left over your head. Straighten up your body your arms go out the side again. Now bend your body right with the right arm goes down in front of the belly and the left arm goes right over your head, repeat 10 times (figure 4).

Month 6 (21st to 25th Week)

This is the period when you start gaining weight faster than ever before. This is because your baby is preparing for the life outside the womb by getting fatter. The baby is also getting stronger and this is why you are able to feel stronger kicks then before.

Week 21: The baby has grown to 27 cm length is now measured from top of the head to the heel. The baby will now weigh about 360 grams. The baby is now gaining weight gradually, adding fat to its body and muscle tissue. The baby's movements are becoming more coordinated, not just jerky twitching movements like before. This is because the muscles are getting stronger. Now the bone marrow starts to make blood cells and the intestines begin to absorb small amounts of sugar from swallowed amniotic fluid.

Week 22: You are now 22 weeks pregnant but foetal age is 20 weeks only, remember the calculation of pregnancy starts from the day of your last menstrual period. The baby is 28 cm long (head to heel) and weighs about 450 grams. The baby reacts even more to loud sounds; recognize not only your voice but the voices of people who are close.

If you're in tune with your body and belly, you will notice that your baby has developed a regular sleeping and waking rhythm. This means your movements and outside noises can wake up the baby. Be careful about this - you don't want to disturb the baby too much as it can affect its nervous system in the future.

The taste buds are now forming on the baby's tongue. This means the baby can taste everything you taste and its taste for food is developing now also. Watch what you eat because in the future your baby is going to like the food you eat now.

My advice at this point is to make sure you eat healthy food and it is balanced.

Week 23: At this point the baby measures over 28 cm and weighs up to 550 grams. The baby's movements are stronger due to it moving more inside the womb and gaining more exercise. The baby turns from side to side and head over heels. The inner ear is now fully developed which controls its sense of balance. This makes the baby sense its position in the womb: whether upside-down or right way up in the womb. The baby can now successfully suck. The pancreas has begun producing insulin, which is important for the breakdown of sugars. Now the baby looks more like a newborn, although it is still very skinny. The baby's fat has not developed much yet to the necessary birth levels. If something happened at this point and the baby was born it would have a 20% chance of survival, but the odds going up with each passing day.

Week 24: Your baby weight is about 650 g now and 30 cm long from head to heel. The baby is gaining weight rapidly now at about 100-150 g per week by building baby fat as well as growing organs, bones and muscles. The baby's face is fully formed and there are a full set of eyelashes, eyebrows, even hair on the head. Right now the hair is white as there is no pigment in the hair just yet. The baby lungs are developing and the cells inside the respiratory tree produce surfactant substance that helps the air sacs inflate and stops them from collapsing.

If born at this stage the baby may well be able to survive with a 50% survival chance at this point. The baby practices breathing by inhaling amniotic fluid into developing lungs. Your little one is still covered with a white protective substance. Some of this substance may still be on the child's skin at birth. The coordination of muscles has improved which allows the baby to suck its thumb easily.

Week 25: Your baby is 34 cm in length and weighs almost 700 grams. The baby is still practicing its breathing but the lungs are still too underdeveloped to function properly. Bones are becoming solid. Hands are fully developed allowing your baby make a fist and clasp objects placed in palm. The skin is still very thin with capillaries forming under the skin. The vocal cord is functional now, leading to occasional hiccups, which you may actually feel. The sexual organs are fully formed and easily visible on ultrasound.

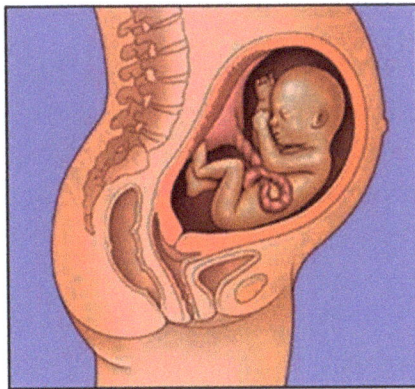

Your baby at 6 month of pregnancy.

Your experiences during the 6th month.

This month is usually associated with an increase in energy. You should have a healthy appetite with little or no nausea, although you may experience some heartburn. Your skin is glowing. Your sex drive may increase or decrease from week to week.

Puffiness of your feet and hands can become more noticeable as the sixth month brings an increase of bodily fluids. The thyroid glands are more active during pregnancy and it can make you sweat more heavily. Some women have leaking breast fluids, which is nothing to worry about. Some women have nose bleeds and bleeding of the gums due to an increase of blood volume during pregnancy.

Many women begin to feel anxious about the health of their baby and what the future will bring. This is perfectly normal. Try to calm yourself with meditation, yoga and by focusing on the positive things.

Sleeping can be a problem as the belly is getting bigger and putting more pressure on your back and organs inside. So try to make yourself comfy in bed as much as possible. There is no such thing as too many pillows when you're pregnant. You may need more pillows under your head and under your feet to keep them elevated at night to prevent swelling. Sleep on your side instead sleeping on your back.

Create a relaxing bedtime routine: nice pleasant rituals before going to bed. Good options to consider are relaxing music, meditation, a warm bath, a massage (or self-massage), light reading or doing relaxing positive affirmations. Avoid caffeine in the afternoon. Before going to bed have a cup of warm milk.

Haemorrhoids in the middle of pregnancy.

Haemorrhoids are very common during pregnancy. Most women have them at a different degree due the hormonal changes and the growing pressure on the internal veins. There are a few things you can do to improve this condition.

First of all you need to follow the right diet and do regular exercise to prevent constipation. Secondly, you need to reduce the pain and look after the painful nodes.

A regular herbal bath or sitz bath can be very helpful. The best herbs are: Lavender, UvaUrsi, Calendula, Rosemary, Sage and Comfrey. Sea salt can be added to the bath for better results. When having a bath try a combination of herbs or use one herb at a time. Test whatever is better for you and if you really like one kind of herb then stick to it.

If you have external haemorrhoids and find wiping after going to the toilet to be painful, try some gentle baby wipes.

To soothe the sting try witch hazel pads or ice packs. Doing Kegels can also ward off haemorrhoids by improving circulation to the area.

Haemorrhoids, if they are not complicated, aren't dangerous just uncomfortable and usually go away after delivery.

Healthy things to do during the 6th month of pregnancy.

The baby is coming soon and you're eagerly awaiting the arrival of your new little one. Labour and birth are strong emotional experiences and you may have some trepidation even panic mixed with excited anticipation. Take a few moments now to feel your body and see if you can identify uncomfortable sensations and notice where you are holding all the apprehension and worry.

What to do in your Pregnancy Diary.

Take your pregnancy diary now and make two lists: one of things you worry about and another one for things you are uncertain or doubtful about.

Acknowledging fears and doubts help dissipate the power they have over you. These feelings of fear and doubt set into motion a kind of physiology of stress, resulting in the releasing of fight-or-flight chemicals into your blood stream. These chemicals can negatively affect your health by constricting your blood vessels that compromises blood circulation in your body. Also the fight-or-flight chemicals lower your pain threshold making you feel the pains and aches in the body more severely.

Fortunately, there is an antidote for this, your breath. Your own breath can bring you to your centre and connect to your mind, body and spirit. It relives the stress and reverses the negative effects of the stress.

Mindfulness of Breath or Breathing for healing.

In this set of exercises you will learn both to relax and con-centrate on your breath. Being able to observe your own breath gives you some form of control over your reactivity and you start to learn self-control, not just relaxation. When you go into labour it is very useful to be able to control your body and your pains during the contractions. This self-control comes from focusing on your own breath.

Let's begin.

Meditation to relieve pregnancy pains and aches.

Sit comfortably, in a chair with your back and neck straight. Take a deep breath in and out. Focus all your attention at the entrance of your nostrils and be aware of the breath coming in, going out: simple breathe, your own breath.

Feel the temperature of the air and be aware that the air is flow-ing continuously at the entrance of your nostrils. Notice if it comes in more through the right or left nostril, if it's deep or shallow, fast or slow.

When you are aware of the incoming and outgoing breath, there is no past or future. You are in the present moment, time almost doesn't exist.

Now imagine that when you inhale, the air goes directly into your belly. Close your eyes and rest your hands on your belly. Allow each intake to enter and fill your belly, enriching your baby. As you breathe out, feel your belly muscles soften and allow each out-breath to be long and slow, releasing tension and tightness from your body.

Your big challenge during this exercise is to withdraw your attention from any ongoing thoughts. Keep breathing consciously. Very alert and attentive. Every time a bad thought arises, see it for what it is. Just a thought. Not the truth, not you. Although there may be true issues within that thought, the thought is just a thought. Learn to see thoughts for what they are without reacting or engaging with them. Without identifying yourself with them. With a degree of detachment.

Now imagine that when you inhale, the air passes the belly and goes down to your pelvic floor. Closing your eyes, breathe in through your pelvic floor and feel your breath flowing up. Allow it to fill your belly, chest, lungs, and brain with nourishing energy. As you exhale, allow your breath to gently release all the tension, softening the muscles all over your body.

Keep practicing. The longer you practice the more changes you will notice in your daily activities, and you will be able to focus better, be less bothered by intrusive thoughts, and develop a degree of self-confidence and self-control.

Every time your mind wanders, do not feel disappointed or defeated. Smilingly bring the awareness back to your breath, mastering your own mind bit by bit progressively. Keep practicing and try to sustain your attention on your breath as long as you can.

Now imagine your breath goes through the body and enters the place where you need healing. It can be a place of pains or aches. It can be your contracting uterus. Relax into the discomfort. Don't try to change it or rid yourself of it. Simply let the pain be. Gently breathe though any tightening, fear, resistance. Loosen your grip.

Focus lightly on the discomfort and feel it completely. As you inhale, breathe all your pain in. Visualise it as a cloud of the black smoke. As the black smoke spreads in your body, it gets purified with your love and compassion. As you exhale imagine this love and compassion as a pink/purple light. Breathe it in again sending it back to the area of pain. Keep doing this: breathing in pain, purify it with love and when you exhale, send the love to the place of pain.

Month 7 (26th to 30th Week)

Welcome to your 3rd and final trimester! During the seventh month of pregnancy, the foetus's senses are awakened. You're in more and more need of rest as the baby continues to develop. This is a time for parents-to-be to prepare for the birth and learn how to communicate with their child.

Week 26: The baby measures 35.5 cm long from the top of the head to the heels and weighs about 800 grams. Your baby's eyes are beginning to open this week. The iris, the coloured part of the eye, still doesn't have much pigmentation so it is too early to tell the baby's eye colour, but the baby can see. You may notice an increased movement now since the baby is even more sensitive to bright light and loud noises. A loud vibrating noise makes it startle and blink. Breathing movements become deeper, but there is no air in the baby's lungs just yet. The baby can calm its self by sucking its thumb; this activity also makes the cheek and jaw muscles stronger. The baby has a predictable routine for sleep and active periods now. But if you are having twins don't expect them to sleep or be awake at the same time.

Week 27: Your baby now weighs about 885 grams and is 36.5 cm in length. The baby is growing rapidly now and gaining weight by building up the fat and muscles tones. The muscle tone is improving and the body is getting bigger. Head and organs also grow in size and the brain continues its rapid development now. The retinas at the back the eyes are developing. The eyes can open, and the baby will notice and may turn its head if you shine a flashlight against your belly. The eyebrows, eyelashes and hair are growing longer every day. The eyes can blink, open and close. The baby can taste your food and respond to spicy food by hiccupping or by kicking. So, remember to eat healthy balanced meals because your baby is developing their tastes for food at this time.

Week 28: The baby's weight has increased to 1000 grams and its length is about 40 cm. By now, your little one can do many things: blinking, coughing, sucking, hiccupping and breathing, but still needs to do more practice on its breathing as the lungs are still developing. It has been proven that by this week the baby has dreams. Brain waves show rapid eye movement (REM) sleep, which means your baby is dreaming. What the baby is dreaming about we will never know. But I would guess it is probably its mum, you. So make sure you show lots of love and affection to your baby and to yourself, as everything you feel and sense, the baby feels and senses.

Week 29: Your baby now weighs about 1250 grams and is around 42 cm in length. The baby's head is growing bigger to accommodate the brain, which is busy developing billions of neurons (brain cells). The eyes are moving in their sockets and the first teeth are starting to develop under the gums. The baby responds to changes in light and different tastes. Research has shown that your baby has formed its preferences or dislikes for particular foods and tastes at this point of development. The baby is putting on weight rapidly now and gaining fat and muscles tissue around the bones. You are likely to feel not only kicks but pokes and jabs from elbows and knees as your womb becomes a bit too tight for its growing body.

Week 30: The baby's length is about 43 cm and your baby's weight is about 1.4 kg. The baby is gaining weight now at a rate of around 200 g per week, getting fatter and is beginning to control its own body temperature. The baby's bones are now mature enough to start producing their own blood supply from their bone marrow, taking over this task from their liver and spleen. From this week your baby develops a new layer of fat called 'brown adipose tissue' (or BAT). This is the kind of fat, that is typically found in

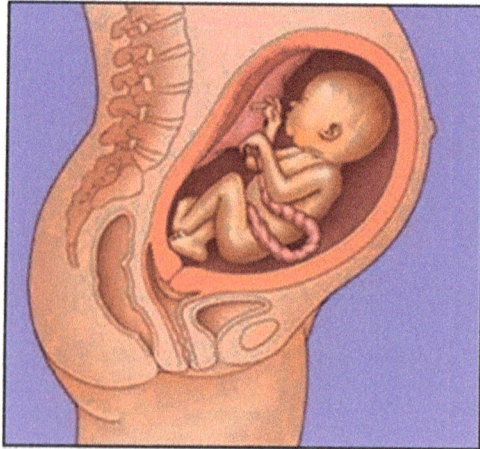

Your baby at the 7th month pregnancy.

hibernating animals. BAT is the baby's main source of heat production after birth; it will keep the baby warm and give it energy to spend when the baby is born. As the fat tissue builds, the wrinkles on your baby's skin start to smooth out. Lanugo (fine hair) continues to cover the baby's body, and will remain there until birth. Your baby's brain has grown and the nervous system is almost mature.

Your experiences during the 7th month of pregnancy.

You must remember that every pregnancy is different and the experiences you have may not be true for other women, during this month. New symptoms may show up or the old ones will persist. You may feel completely perfect and full of energy and that is great!

But for reference here is what women generally feel during the 7th month.

- Your uterus begins to tighten and relax at odd moments or an irregular intervals. These are painless contractions, called Braxton Hicks contractions. These contractions are practicing for birth. You don't need to worry about them, just relax more and stay in tune with your belly.
- You may easily get out of breath just doing everyday tasks. This is normal, because the uterus is growing and putting a lot of pressure on your lungs. Get some rest. Practice the breathing technique or do meditation or yoga.
- Vulval varicose veins: These veins appear between the 7th and 8th month, and start off with feelings of heaviness or itching. They can be painful during sexual intercourse but often subside 3 to 4 months after giving birth. Avoid hot baths and strong spices such as cayenne, mustard, black pepper, hot sauces and curry.

- Water retention and swelling: It's normal for the ankles, legs and face to swell. A woman's body contains more water when she is pregnant. The best thing you can do is drink lots of water (1.5 litres per day) to drain your tissue properly. To avoid swelling, avoid wearing clothes that are tight around your ankles and wrists. If swelling occurs suddenly, contact your doctor as soon as possible as this could be a sign of a kidney problem.
- Back pain: This gets worse during the last few months of pregnancy. Adopting correct posture when sitting or standing and doing the stretching exercises we have covered earlier will offer relief. Meditation and other alternative methods of pain relieve can be a great help at this time. Gentle exercise like swimming or walking will help you get back on form.
- Emotionally you may feel exited and anxious at the same time. You may have strange and vivid dreams. Your absent-mindedness continues.

Important thing to know at the 7th month of pregnancy.

Towards the end of the pregnancy, you should pay more attention to having a good rest. Sleeping problems are frequent because lying down becomes more and more uncomfortable. Also the thoughts of giving birth may occupy your mind and keeping you awake at night.

During this time relaxation, meditation and yoga become indispensable tools to cope with pregnancy problems. Taking regular light naps and sleep in a freshly aired room can help to feel stronger and cope with tiredness. If you feel like changing places to sleep, then do so: the sofa can sometimes be more comfortable than your bed.

During this time don't be shy about asking for help with housework or shopping. To avoid the risks of premature birth, keep your lifestyle as stress-free as you can. Continue to do regular exercise as it is important to keep yourself fit and strong, also it prepares you for a safer labour and giving birth.

You should now start attending antenatal classes. In these classes you will learn what happens during childbirth, how to handle the pain, plus breathing techniques and relaxation exercises. It's important to go to these classes because childbirth does require preparation! The more you learn about your body during pregnancy the more in tune with your body you'll become. Listening to your body helps to prevent major problems and helps you to cope with your little one later.

During the 7th month you should be aware of premature labour. Although the changes of the baby arriving early are small, it helps if you know the signs of premature labour and be able to detect it early. Early detection can change the outcome and give you a good chance to carry the pregnancy to term.

Premature labour or warning signs and symptoms:

- Regular painful contractions in your uterus every 10 minutes or more often.
- Menstrual like cramps that may feel like gas pains, with or without diarrhoea, nausea or indigestion.
- Constant backache that changing positions and other comfort measures don't ease.
- Increased pressure in your pelvis or vagina
- Increased vaginal discharge with or without vaginal bleeding
- Leaking fluids from your vagina.
- Less movement or kicking by your baby

The fact is that the majority of women, who have symptoms of premature labour, do not deliver early. But detecting the signs early will help your doctor to proceed with preventive measures and help you to continue with the pregnancy.

Healthy things to do during the 7th month.

In the seventh month, your baby can hear your voice, your heartbeat and even the voices of your family clearly. Your baby's senses are awakened during this month. So, don't forget to share music, conversation, and even books with your baby. Relax and meditate tuning into your belly and sending the baby your love. Always be sure to say lots of nice things and make other people like your husband or the father of the baby do the same.

Progressive muscle relaxation technique for pregnancy and birth.

Progressive muscle relaxation techniques have been used to combat stress, fear, anxiety, insomnia, evenchronic pain. This method can also be applied to pregnancy as well as natural childbirth. Through ongoing practice you can quickly learn to recognize and tell the difference between a tensed muscle and a completely relaxed one.

Being aware of this you can then apply physical muscular relaxation techniques at the first signs of stress. Doing physical relaxation method scan gives you mental peace in most situations, even when you experience pains and aches due to pregnancy and giving birth.

Doing progressive muscle relaxation techniques is a two-step process. First is tightening a particular muscle or a muscle group and then releasing the tension. Once you let go the tension, you then focus your attention on how the muscle or muscle group feels as the tension eases away. It is not hard to do and mastery of this technique can be achieved in approximately 10-20 minutes of practice per day. Progressive muscle relaxation techniques are usually undertaken in a set sequence:

Hands
Forearms
Arms
Head (forehead, scalp, eyes, mouth and jaw, tongue and lips)
Neck
Shoulders
Lungs
Belly
Legs
Feet and toes
Relaxation of the whole body
Let's start doing progressive muscle relaxation now...

Meditation: Progressive muscle relaxation technique for pregnancy.

Begin to relax as you take a few slow deep breaths, deep with your stomach not your chest. As you let the rest of your body relax, clench your fists and bend them back at the wrist, tighter and tighter. Yes, keep breathing and feel the tension in your fists and forearms. Now relax. Feel the looseness in your hands and forearms. Notice the contrast between being relaxed and when they were tense?

Now bend your elbows and tense your biceps. Tense them as hard as you can and observe the feeling of tautness. Let your arms drop down now and relax. Feel the difference between the tension and relaxation.

Now turn your attention to your head, and wrinkle your forehead. Yes, as tight as you can. Feel the tension in the forehead and scalp. Now relax and smooth it out. Imagine your entire forehead and scalp becoming smooth and at rest.

Now frown and notice the strain spreading throughout your forehead. Keep breathing, and let go. Relax: allow your brow to become smooth again.

Squeeze your eyes closed. Tighter: keep breathing, and relax your eyes. Let them remained closed, gently and comfortably.

Now open your mouth wide and feel tension in your jaw. Relax your jaw. When the jaw is relaxed your lips will be slightly parted. Notice the contrast between the tension and relaxation.

Now press your tongue against the roof of your mouth. Experience the ache at the back of your mouth. Keep breathing through your nose. Now relax.

Pout your lips now, purse them into an "O" shape: now relax your lips. Feel the relaxation in your forehead, scalp, eyes, jaw, tongue, and lips. Let go more and more.

Now roll your head slowly around your neck, feeling the point of tension shifting as your head moves. Then slowly roll your head the other way. Keep breathing and relax, allowing your head to return to a comfortable upright position.

Now shrug your shoulders. Bring your shoulders up towards your ears. Hold it: now drop your shoulders back down and feel the relaxation spreading through your neck, throat, and shoulders. Shrug the shoulders again. Hold it, keep breathing: now drop your shoulders and relax. Feel the sensation of being relaxed in your shoulders.

Now breathe in and fill up your lungs completely and hold your breath. Experience the tension. Now exhale and let your chest become loose. Try again filling your lungs completely and hold your breath. Experience the tension; you might even feel sensations in your cheeks and face: now exhale. Continue relaxing, letting your breath come freely and gently. Notice the tension draining out of your muscles with each exhalation.

Next, tighten your belly and hold. Keep breathing: feel the tension and relax. Now place your hands on your belly. Breathe deeply into your stomach pushing your hands up: hold and relax. Feel the contrast between relaxation and the tension as the air rushes out. Now try doing it again.

Now arch your back, without straining. Keep the rest of your body as relaxed as possible. Focus on the tension in your lower back: now relax. Let the tension dissolve away.

Now, tighten your buttocks and thighs. Keep breathing and feel the tension: now relax and feel the difference. Try doing it again. Tighten your buttocks and thighs. Stronger, tighter, keep breathing, feel the tension: now relax.

Now straighten and tense your legs and curl your toes downwards. Keep breathing. Experience the tension: now relax. Again, straighten and tense your legs, but this time bend your toes towards your face: tighter and tighter, keep breathing, feel the tension: now relax.

Try and feel the comfortable warmth and heaviness of deep relaxation throughout your entire body as you continue to breathe slowly and deeply. You can relax even more as you move up through your body, letting go all of the last bits of tension in your body.

Now try to relax even more? Start with your feet; relax your feet. Move up and relax your ankles. Relax your calves. Relax your shins. Relax your knees, your thighs, and buttocks. Let the relaxation spread through your belly, to your lower back, to your chest. Let go more and more. Feel the relaxation deepening in your shoulders, in your arms, and in your hands, let it go deeper and deeper. Notice the feeling of looseness and relaxation in your neck, your jaw, your face, and your scalp.

Continue to breathe, slowly and deeply, down in your stomach. Your entire body is comfortably loose and relaxed, calm, and rested…

Progressive muscle relaxation technique can be successfully used for management of pains and aches during pregnancy as well as pain control during labour. For the best effect you must practice this technique daily. Only with practice you can achieve good control of your body.

Month 8 (31st to 35th Week)

During this month the baby is gaining weight and growing very fast, these changes are becoming quite visible on the mother's body as well. Your belly becomes more visible and larger with each and every day. Your muscle cramps become more intense as the uterus pushes all muscles and skin covering the abdomen. This is a time when you need to be sure that you are taking care of yourself and not trying to prove something to yourself or your family. Get plenty of rest, eat healthy, meditate, do yoga, walk and exercise according to your abilities.

Week 31: The baby's weight is around 1.8 kg and length around 42-46 cm. The baby is still growing and should more than double its weight again between now and birth. Almost all the organs are developed now and working. The baby is passing water from the bladder. Muscle tissue and fat are growing fast. The brain is producing new neurons (brain cells) and creating new connections between them. The eyes have now completely opened and are responding to light and darkness. The lungs continue to mature, producing increasing amounts of 'surfactant', the substance which keeps airways moist and helping the alveoli (airway sacks) to expand efficiently for breathing. If born at 31 to 32 weeks, babies have about a 95% chance of survival but most of them still need to be cared for in an intensive care nursery.

Week 32: The baby is about 45 cm long and weighs about 1.9 kg. During this time the baby sleeps most of the day. The uterus is getting to be a small space for the baby to move around, so you may have noticed a decrease in your baby's movements. The baby is still trying to move frequently but it just does not have enough room. The baby will turn its head from side to side and move its hands.

In boys, the testicles will be descending from the groin down into his scrotum. In girls, the clitoris is now relatively prominent. Your baby's skin is no longer see-through as more and more fat accumulates under the skin.

Week 33: The baby inside you now weighs about 2 kg and can be 46-48 cm long. The head diameter is about 8.5 cm and it is palpable above your pubic bone. Most babies take a 'head down' position around this time and stay this way until they are born. The baby is still growing fat and muscles are becoming bigger and bigger. The baby taste becomes more sophisticated, and now your baby can determine the difference between sweet and sour when it swallows the surrounded amniotic fluid. Your baby is drinking about half a litre of amniotic fluid a day and urinating the same amount. Lanugo (early hair) is disappearing and being replaced by actual hair. The nails of your baby are now long enough to reach to the tip of the fingers or beyond and may need trimming as soon as the baby is born. Babies can even scratch their faces while still in uterus. The immune system continues to develop and antibodies are being passed from you to your baby. These antibodies will protect the baby from germs.

Week 34: The baby is now 48-50 cm top of head to the heel and weighs about 2.4 kg. Your baby has now an excellent chance of survival outside the womb as all the organs have developed, but the growth still continues. The baby's position should be upside down because the baby is preparing for birth. In boys the testicles are going down from the abdomen to the scrotum. The immune system is developing intensely during this time as antibodies continue to cross the placenta, giving the baby more immunity against infections.

Week 35: The baby is about 47-50 cm from top of head to the heel and weighs almost 2.7 Kg. Because the baby is getting so big for the space in your uterus, you may notice baby isn't moving around as much. Most babies gain about 250 grams per week at this time of pregnancy. The legs and arms are becoming fatter and muscle is developing more. The baby's fat is now needed to regulate their body temperature. But it is still not enough fat to keep it warm if outside of uterus. If born now, the baby would need to stay in an incubator at least for some time. The kidneys are fully developed and the liver can also process some waste products. Now, the baby's reflexes become coordinated: and baby is turning its head, grasping, and responding to sounds, light and touch.

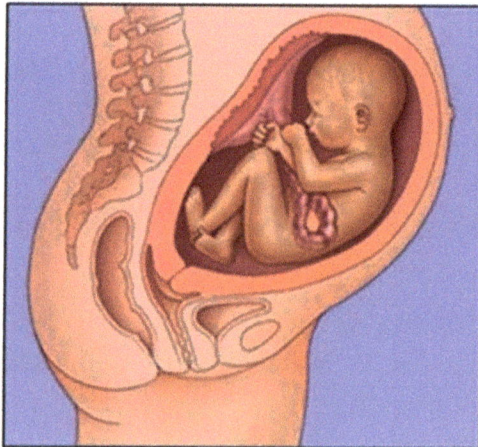

Your baby at 8 months pregnant.

Your experiences during the 8th month of pregnancy.

During the 8th month of pregnancy you will be feeling regular strong movements from the baby. You will begin to feel bony parts, such as heels, knees and elbows sticking out periodically. As the baby pushes up on your lungs, you may feel short of breath. This is normal and will get better as the baby drops into the birth position. Many symptoms from earlier months continue:

- Occasional headaches, faintness or dizziness.
- Heartburn, bloating and indirections.
- Nasal congestion and occasional nosebleeds.
- Haemorrhoids.
- Increased constipation.
- Sensitive gums.
- Leg cramps.
- Varicose veins on legs and other parts of the body.
- Itchy abdomen (because the skin is stretched)
- Difficulty in sleeping.
- Increasing clumsiness.
- Enlarged and tender breasts.
- Uterus contractions (Braxton Hicks)
- Colostrum leaking from nipples.
- Backaches.
- Mild swelling of the feet, ankles and occasionally of the hands and face.

Emotionally you maybe experience trepidation about becoming a parent. Excitement and anxiety at the same time. All these feelings are normal for this part of your pregnancy.

Preparing for Birth Exercises.
Pelvic Tilt.

Performing pelvic tilt exercises during pregnancy is essential in order to keep mobility in the low back, hips and pelvis. Pelvic tilt exercises also help maintain abdominal muscle tone and provide a mild low back stretch, which can help ease the lower back pain and discomfort that often accompanies pregnancy, particularly in the last two trimesters.

You can do pelvic tilt exercises standing, lying on your back, or kneeling.

Standing position for the pelvic tilt:

- Stand straight with your back to the wall and relax your spine.
- Place your feet shoulder width apart.
- Use your hands to find a small arch in your low back so there is space between your lower back and the wall.
- The back of your head, shoulder blades, and tailbone should be touching the wall.
- Take a deep breath, and as you exhale slowly press your lower back towards the wall as your tailbone slides down the wall.
- With your next exhale, slide your tailbone up the wall and create an arch in the lower back.
- Perform at least 5 to 10 repetitions of each pelvic tilt.

Kneeling position for the pelvic tilt:

- Kneel on all fours. Your hands should be directly under your shoulders, knees directly under your hips, spine neutral.
- INHALE: Gently tilt the pelvis forward, dropping hips toward the floor.
- EXHALE: Pull in your abs as you tilt your pelvis backward, up toward the ceiling to complete one rep.
- Repeat for 10-15 repetitions, 1-2 sets.

Lying on the back the pelvic tilt:
- Lie on your back with your knees bent.
- Inhale through your nose and tighten your stomach and buttock muscles.
- Flatten the small of your back against the floor and allow your pelvis to tilt upward.
- Hold for a count of five as you exhale slowly.
- Relax and repeat.
- **Note:** DO NOT arch your back, bulge your abdomen or push with your feet to obtain this motion!

Yoga exercises and stretching.

Here is a short complex of yoga exercises for those of you who haven't done yoga before but want to start now at the 8th month of pregnancy.

1. Sit on a chair. Straighten your back and neck. Centre yourself by taking a few deep breaths. Meditate for a few minutes focusing just on your breath until you feel completely relaxed in your body. When you become relaxed, do the Kegels exsercise 10 times. Tighten your pelvic floor muscles, hold the contraction for five seconds, and then relax for five seconds. Try it four or five times in a row. Work up to keeping the muscles contracted for 10 seconds at a time, and relaxing for 10 seconds between contractions.

2. Sit crossed-legged on the floor; put your hands on your lap. Lift the right arm up and stretch the right side of your body for 10 seconds. Then, do the same with your left arm. Breathe in and out. Focus just on your breath and feel the sensations in your body when stretching. If any thoughts arise, just gently push them away. Repeat 10-20 times.

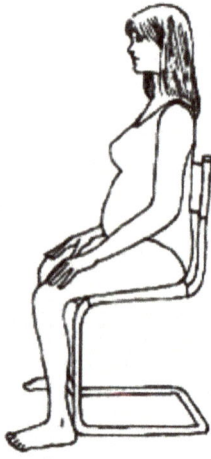

1

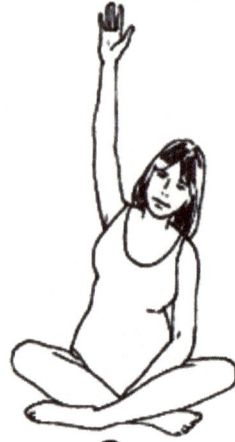

2

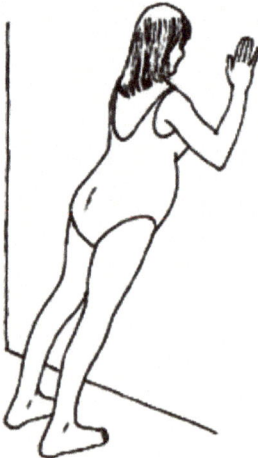

3

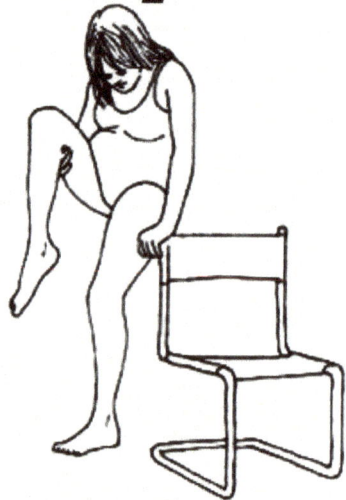

4

3. Stand 30-40 cm from the wall. Your feet should be shoulder width apart. Bend your elbow in a 90 degree angle. Palms are towards the wall. Move your body to the wall keeping your both feet firmly on the floor. Then, push away from the wall. Repeat 10 times.

4. Stand at a chair (or a table) and hold it with one hand. With the other hand hold the same side leg below the knee. Pull the leg up, stretching the thigh and buttocks. Change sides. Repeat 10 times with each side.

Perineal massage.

To prepare yourself for childbirth you can try perineal massage. Perineum is the area around your vagina. Daily perineal massage may increase the area's ability to stretch, leading to less need for an episiotomy and fewer natural tears. The best time to start this massage is about 34th week of pregnancy.

While you massage, you can practice relaxing the muscles in your perineum. This can help you prepare for the stretching, burning feeling you may have when your baby's head is born. Relaxing this area during birth can help prevent tearing.

How to do the perineal massage?

1. Wash your hands well, and keep your fingernails short. Relax in a private place with your knees bent.

2. Lubricate your thumbs and the perineal tissues. Use a lubricant such as vitamin E oil or almond oil, or any vegetable oil used for cooking—like olive oil. You may also try a water-soluble jelly, such as K-Y jelly, or your body's natural vaginal lubricant. Do not use baby oil, mineral oil, or petroleum jelly.

3. Place your thumbs about 1 to 1.5 inches inside your vagina. Press down (toward the anus) and to the sides until you feel a slight burning, stretching sensation. Hold that position for 1 or 2 minutes.

4. With your thumbs, slowly massage the lower half of the vagina using a "U" shaped movement. Concentrate on relaxing your muscles. This is a good time to practice slow, deep breathing techniques.

Massage your perineal area slowly for 10 minutes each day. After 1 to 2 weeks, you should notice more stretchiness and less burning in your perineum.

Partners: If your partner is doing the perineal massage, follow the same basic instructions, above. However, your partner should use his or her index fingers to do the massage (instead of thumbs). The same side-to-side, U-shaped, downward pressure method should be used. Good communication is important for the massage to be effective.

Note: make sure not to damage the perineum during the massage. It should be done in a gentle careful manner. Bruising and hurting the area will do more damage than good. This is one of the disadvantages of the perineal massage if the area gets damaged during the massage.

Month 9 (36th to 40th Week)

Congratulations! You are now in the last month of pregnancy. You will be able to hold your baby in your own arms any time now. It is only a matter of days before the much-anticipated day comes: the day when your baby is born. You should be proud of yourself for all that you have endured over the past nine months. Preparation is the key, and will make a huge difference to how you experience labor and manage the pain. Make sure that you take the time and create the mental space to visualize what is about to happen.

> **Week 36:** Your little one weighs about 2.7 kg and is about 49-51 cm long. Between now and birth they may gain about an ounce (30 g) a day. Right now most of baby's organs and systems are equipped for life outside the uterus. Baby continues gaining weight as fat deposits and is forming creases in the neck and wrists. Your baby

is almost ready, the kidneys and the liver have begun processing some waste products, and the only organ still to mature is the lungs. The baby may drop into the birth canal any time soon.

Week 37: The baby is considered "at term" and measures about 50-51 cm from head to heels and weighs about 3 kg. The head diameter is over 9cm. Although the baby is completely ready to live outside the uterus he/she is still growing and putting on weight. The baby is practicing his/her skills: simulating breathing by inhaling and exhaling amniotic fluid, sucking on his/her thumb, blinking, and turning from side to side.

Week 38: The baby is about 50-53 cm and weighs about 3.4 kg. The baby development is complete. He/she may have a full head of hair now, an inch or more long. Most of the lanugo (early hair) has disappeared, but you may see some on the upper back and shoulders when he or she arrives. The vernixcaseosa, the whitish substance that covered baby is almost gone .The baby swallows the lanugo and exterior coating, along with other secretions, and stores them in the bowel. These will become your infant's first bowel movement, a blackish waste called meconium. The lungs are producing more and more surfactant, which will prevent air sacs from collapsing when your baby starts to breath.

Week 39: The average baby is about 50-53 cm and weighs about 3 -3.5 kg. The head is about 10 cm in diameter. The baby's head has dropped into your pelvis, making your breathing a bit easier. He/she is in its final birth position and is ready come out any time. You still feel kicking and punching but much lower in your abdomen. The baby's brain is still developing and this process will continue during the first three years of life. His/her pink skin has now turned white-milky colour (the pigmentation doesn't occur until later after birth, for this reason most newborn babies are light colour, even those from dark skinned parents). Most newborn babies from white-skinned parents have blue eyes and their true eye colour may not reveal itself for months after the birth. Most African and Asian babies usually have dark grey or brown eyes at birth, which will change to their true brown or black colours in about 6-12 months after the birth.

Week 40: Congratulations! Your baby is full term and weighs anything between 2.7 – 4 kg and is about 48-56 cm in lengths. The weight and size can depend on many factors: constitutional, genetic, environmental and etc. All the baby systems are developed and ready to go. He/she is getting ready for birth and is settling into the fetal position with its head down against the birth canal, its legs tucked up to its chest, and its knees against its nose. The head bones are soft and flexible to make it easy to pass through the birth canal. The umbilical cord is strong and tense from the rapid blood flow. He/she will continue to kick and punch although it will move lower in your abdomen.

Many pregnancies proceed past the 40 weeks mark; and this is Ok as long as it doesn't go over the 42nd week.

Week 41-42: You didn't think that you would still be pregnant past your due date. The biggest reason, that it seems that you go overdue is a miscalculation of your original conception date. Doctors count the start of your pregnancy from the first day of your last menstrual period but the actual conception occurs much later. The exact date of conception is difficult to pinpoint and that's where a mistake of your due date is coming from.

Generally, the longer your pregnancy goes, the bigger your baby gets. Your doctor must be watching the size of your baby very closely. If the baby gets too big - it won't pass through the birth canal and a Caesarean section may be required. If your baby is still in the normal range then chances are your doctor will let you go into labour on your own.

Some post-term babies are not different in appearance than term infants. But general signs of post-term babies are: dry, loose and peeling skin; long fingernails and toenails; thick, long head hair; and thin arms and legs. As the baby a little older, he/she may also be more alert than the average newborn.

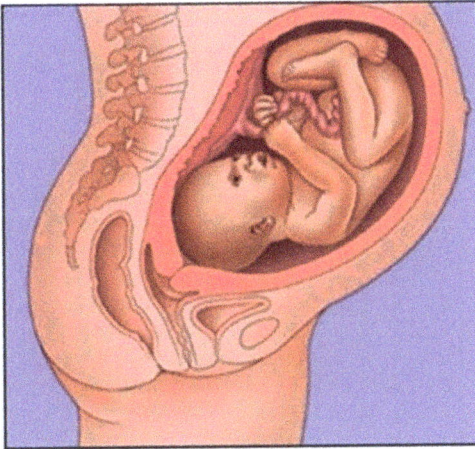

Your baby during 9 month of pregnancy.

Your experiences during the 9th month.

Your body goes through changes throughout your entire pregnancy, but during the last month, it all becomes very noticeable. Some physical symptoms you may experience, include:

- Your weight remains pretty constant but some women actually report dropping one or two pounds during these last weeks, but the change may not be very noticeable.
- Body aches can become bothersome: back aches, tingly legs and hands, belly aches.
- Increased urination still bothers you.
- Swelling on feet and hands continues.
- Skin blotches may become even more obvious.
- Hemorrhoid and varicose veins are still present.
- Breathing becomes easier as the baby has dropped into a birth canal and kicks in the ribs aren't as frequent as they were.
- Breasts produce colostrum in higher amounts.
- Braxton Hicks contractions become a little more frequent in the first weeks and very intense as the due date approaches. However, they're not painful until pregnancy week 40, when these contractions turn into real labor contractions, announcing childbirth.

Back pain during the last trimester.

Back pain is common during pregnancy and it is related to a number of factors. One of them is increased hormones. The hormones during pregnancy make ligaments in the pelvic area soften and the joints become looser in preparation for childbirth. These changes may affect the support of your back and it becomes painful. Additional weight can also affect your back support. The other reason for a backache is shifting center of gravity. It moves forward as your uterus grows. Poor posture, excessive standing, and bending over can trigger or escalate the back pain. Stress usually finds the weak spot in the body, so you may experience an increase in back pain during stressful periods.

Here are a few tips to reduce the back pain during pregnancy:

- Physical exercises that support and help strengthen the back and abdomen. These exercises are walking, swimming, dancing and aerobic. Do it for 20-30 min at least 4-5 days a week (preferably every day). Take care to exercise at a mild to moderate level, but not to the point of exhaustion.
- When you have to pick up something from the floor squat instead of bending over.
- Avoid high heels and other shoes that do not provide adequate support.
- Get a comfortable sleeping position. The best sleeping position is on your left side with your knees bent up and two or more pillows placed between your knees. This position will alleviate pressure and strain from your lower back. Sleeping on this side will also increase the amount of nutrients and blood that reach your baby. Avoid sleeping on your back.
- Wear a support belt under your lower abdomen.
- Get plenty of rest. Elevating your feet is also good for your back.
- Water massage: turn the shower head to pulsating and enjoy the back massage.
- Alternate ice or heat to your back muscles. Use an ice pack for 15 min, followed by a heating pad for 15 minutes applying those to your back muscles.
- Braces or support devices can be helpful to relieve the back pain.
- Meditation, relaxation and yoga are considered to be the best treatments for back pain by many people who practise these exercises.

How to sit correctly to support your back.

Good posture is needed to support your back while pregnant. There
are several steps you can take to
maintain good posture and proper
body mechanics while sitting.

Sit up with your back straight and
your shoulders back. Your buttocks
should touch the back of your chair.

Sit with a back support (such as
a small, rolled-up towel or a lumbar
roll) at the curve of your back.

Distribute your body weight
evenly on both hips.

Keep your hips and knees at a right angle (use a foot rest or
stool if necessary). Your legs should not be crossed and your feet
should be flat on the floor.

Try to avoid sitting in the same position for more than 30 minutes. At work, adjust your chair height and workstation so you can
sit up close to your desk. Rest your elbows and arms on your chair
or desk, keeping your shoulders relaxed.

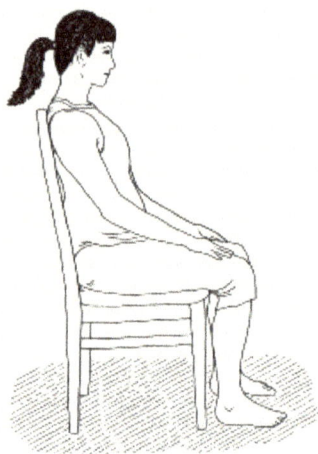

Healthy things to do during the 9th month of pregnancy.

Daily meditation, yoga and relaxation are the best things you
can do this time to clear your mind and ward off anxiety. Continue
your birth preparation by regular practicing of breathing techniques, muscles stretching and relaxation.

Choose low impact forms of exercise. During the second and
third trimesters of pregnancy, the body releases a hormone called
"relaxin" that loosens your ligaments and joints in preparation for
labor. While softer ligaments facilitate delivery of the baby, it puts

you at higher risk for injury or falling down when you exercise. For your final month, choose gentle exercises such as swimming or walking, which do not put undue stress on your joints. Other popular forms of exercise for the ninth month include prenatal yoga, squats, stretches and pelvic tilts.

What can these exercises do for you?

- These exercises improve blood circulation and minimize the problems of water retention and edema.
- Reduce the anxiety, stress and improve sleep.
- Increase adaptability to the new situations by strengthening the nervous system.
- Strengthen muscles and joints.
- Regulate blood pressure during pregnancy by improving circulation.
- Improve posture and help easing back problems.
- Help to stretch many ligaments throughout the pelvic, hip and leg areas, which ease labor pain.
- Strengthens the abdominal muscles which take part in pushing the baby through the birth canal.

Pre-birth exercises.

Squats

It may not be the most elegant position, but squatting is a time-honoured way of preparing for and giving birth. This exercise strengthens your thighs and helps open your pelvis.

- Stand facing the back of a chair with your feet slightly more than hip-width apart, toes pointed outward. You can hold the back of the chair for support.

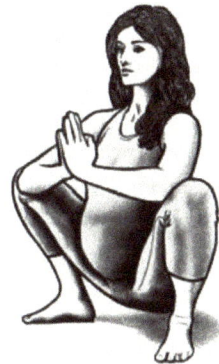

- Contract your abdominal muscles, lift your chest, and relax your shoulders. Then start lowering your tailbone toward the floor as though you were sitting down on a chair. Distribute your weight on your feet, find your balance and maintain squatting position.
- Take a deep breath in and then exhale, pushing into your legs to rise to a standing position.
- Repeat 5-7 times or as much as you feel comfortable.

Kegels

You probably have started doing Kegels in the beginning of your pregnancy. But now Kegels become more and more important as you are preparing for delivery. They can do miracles if you do them regularly: they can protect you from many women health problems related to childbirth.

To remind you, Kegel exercises are small internal contractions of the pelvic floor muscles that support your urethra, bladder, uterus, and rectum. Strengthening your pelvic floor muscles improves circulation in your rectal and vaginal area, helping to keep hemorrhoids at bay, prevent urination problems and speedup the recovery after an episiotomy or tears. There's even some evidence suggesting that strong pelvic floor muscles may shorten the pushing stage of labour.

To do Kegels just tighten the muscles around your vagina as if trying to interrupt the flow of urine when going to the bathroom. Hold for a count of four, then release. Repeat ten times. Try to do Kegels as often as you can.

Tailor or Cobbler Pose

This position can help open your pelvis and loosen your hip joints in preparation for birth. It can also improve your posture and ease tension in your lower back.

- Sit up straight against a wall with the soles of your feet touching each other (sit on a folded towel if that's more comfortable for you).
- Gently press your knees down and away from each other, but don't force them.
- Stay in this position for as long as you're comfortable.

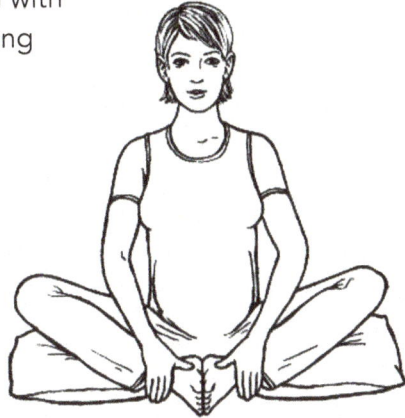

Dromedary Droop or Angry Cat.

This exercise is helpful to prepare you for birth and also to relive back pain.

Starting Position

Start on your hands and knees with both approximately shoulder width apart. Keep your back straight and in a neutral position, do not allow your back to sag. Keep your neck straight also.

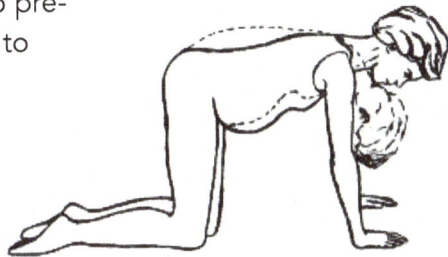

Action

Bump or arch your back up like a cat, allowing your head to drop down (chin to chest). Tighten your abdominal muscles and buttocks during this movement as well. Return to the Starting Position. Repeat 10-15 repetitions for 1-2 sets.

This exercise strengthens your body, your back and is very useful before and during labour.

False Labour, Pre-Labour or Real Labour?

False labour.

Sometimes, in the end of pregnancy, the painless Braxton Hicks contractions that you may have been feeling since mid-pregnancy become more rhythmic, and even painful, possibly fooling you into thinking you're in labour. But unlike true labour, this so-called false labour doesn't cause significant, progressive dilation of your cervix, and the contractions don't grow consistently longer, stronger, and closer together. These contractions are preparations for the labour but not a true labour.

It is hard to tell the difference between false labour and the early stages of true labour. These things might help you sort it out:

False labour	True labour
Contractions are unpredictable. They come at irregular intervals and vary in length and intensity.	Contractions are predictable. They come in a certain interval and with a certain length.
The pain from the contractions is more likely to be centred in your lower abdomen.	The pain start in your lower back and wrap around to your abdomen.
Contractions usually subside when you start or stop an activity or change position.	Contractions will persist and progress no matter what you do.

What should you do if you start having contractions?

If you're not yet 37 weeks, you should contact your doctor immediately to rule out preterm labour. After 37 weeks, you can sit out the contractions (whether false or from true early labour) at home and see what develops, unless your practitioner has advised you otherwise.

Pre-labour.

In a few weeks before labour begins, your body starts producing hormones that prepare you to give birth. This process is called pre-labour and it is characterised by the beginning of cervical effacement and dilation of the cervix. These findings can be confirmed by your practitioner on examination. The signs that you may notice include:

Pre-labour signs	Comments
Dropping of the baby.	It starts somewhere between 2-4 weeks before the labour.
Backache and period pain.	Many women will feel lower backache, or a dull throbbing pain, similar to period cramping. It can come and go, or it may be there all the time.
Loss of the mucous plug.	During pregnancy, your cervix secretes mucous which forms a thick mucus plug. The purpose of the plug is to prevent any bacteria getting into the uterus. During the last couple of weeks of pregnancy or up until labour itself, the plug will start to come away so the baby can pass through the cervix. It may look like a thick glob of stringy mucous, thicker than what you would see with normal vaginal secretions. Some women do not even notice their plug expelling as there is already an increase in normal cervical mucus due to hormones.

Bloody show.	As your cervix begins to open, you might notice a thick, stringy, blood-tinged discharge from your vagina. This is known as bloody show.
Braxton Hicks contractions	These become more frequent than usual.
Diarrhoea.	Many expecting moms experience bouts of diarrhoea before labour due to the constant hormonal changes that are happening in her body. Others suffer because Mother Nature is preparing the body for all the pushing she must do to give birth.

Real labour signs:

1. Contractions

When you think you are in true labour, start timing your contractions. To do this, write down the time each contraction starts and stops or have someone do it for you. The time between contractions includes the length or duration of the contraction and the minutes in between the contractions. In real labour:

- Contractions come at regular intervals and last about 30-70 seconds. As time progresses, they get closer together.
- Contractions continue despite movement or changing positions.
- Contractions steadily increase in strength.
- Contractions usually start in the lower back and move to the front of the abdomen.

2. Your water breaks.

When the fluid-filled amniotic sac surrounding your baby ruptures, fluid leaks from your vagina. And whether it comes out in a large gush or a small trickle, you should call your doctor or midwife.

Natural ways to Induce Labour.

Natural ways to induce labour may be chosen for a few reasons:

- Your due date has come but there are no signs of labour.
- You are overdue.
- You want to avoid invasive medical ways to induce labour.

It is good to remember that your baby will come out when he/ she is good and ready but the longer you wait the bigger the baby gets. A big baby is difficult to deliver by a normal vaginal delivery. So, if you want to avoid this complication you can try to induce labour naturally.

Note: Always ask your practitioner about the safety of natural labour induction in your particular situation.

1. Nipple stimulation can help with labour induction. You can start gentle rubbing or rolling of the nipple to encourage the beginning of contractions. Nipple stimulation makes your body to produce oxytocin, a hormone that causes contractions. The usual recommendation is to stimulate the breasts for an hour, three times a day, spending 15 minutes continually stimulating one breast and then alternating to the other breast for 15 minutes until the hour is up.

2. Castor oil. It's a laxative which can stimulate your bowels (by causing spasms in the intestines) and, in turn, irritate your uterus and cause it to start contracting.

   Warning: you can have a bad case of diarrhoea (something you probably want to avoid this close to childbirth). So, it is better if you talk with your practitioner before you take it.

3. Sex and especially orgasm stimulate the uterus and cause it to start contracting. Sperm contains prostaglandins —

hormones that can help thin and dilate the cervix, ripening it for delivery. What's more, an orgasm releases the hormone oxytocin, which can trigger contractions.

4. Homeopathy. Pulsatilla and Caulophyllum are two commonly used homeopathic remedies used to stimulate labour.

5. Eating pineapple. Pineapple contains the enzyme bromelain which is thought to help to soften the cervix and so bring on labour.

6. Herbal: blue cohosh and black cohosh are used to stimulate uterus and bring on labour.

   Warning: don't use these before 39th week of pregnancy.

7. Spicy food and curry can sometimes bring on labour. The theory is that it stimulates the guts and bowel and so encourages the uterus to get going by that means.

8. Acupuncture. Acupuncture involves the insertion of very fine needles into specific points of the body. According to tradiitonal Chinese philosophy, this stimulates the energy within the body to act on a specific organ function or system.

9. Red raspberry leaf. Raspberry leaf can be taken as a tea or in tablet form. It is often mentioned alongside other methods for bringing on labour.

10. Evening primrose oil can help the cervix thin and dilate and prepare it for labour. You can take evening primrose oil capsules, or rub the oil onto your cervix during the last weeks of pregnancy. You can even insert the capsules into your vagina. But be sure to talk to your practitioner before trying evening primrose oil — women with placenta previa should stay away from this herb.

11. Walking helps draw the baby down into your pelvis (thanks to gravity and the swaying of your hips). The pressure of your baby's head pressing down on the cervix from the

inside stimulates the release of oxytocin, which can bring on labour. Also, the gravity itself can help to make the baby want to come out.

Acupressure points to induce labour.

Stimulating of special acupressure points can be helpful to induce labour naturally and avoid medical stimulation. There are a few points which are normally used for this.

LI4 (Hegu point).

It is located in the webbing between your index finger and thumb. It is deep inside the webbing, between the first and second metacarpal bones.

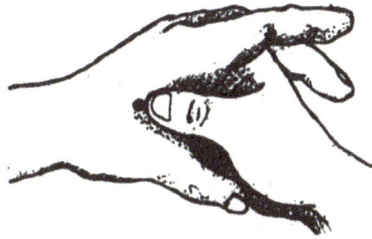

Pinch the area between the index finger and thumb of your opposite hand. Rub your fingers in a circular motion for 30 to 60 seconds. Stop for a few minutes and start rubbing again until you feel a contraction start. Continue rubbing the area between contractions until contractions become regular.

SP6 (San-yin-jiao) point.

Reach down towards one or both of your ankles. You can use acupressure on one leg at a time or on both legs at once.

Place your hand on your leg directly above your ankle. The san-yin-chiao acupressure point will be on the lateral tibia, at the level of your index finger.

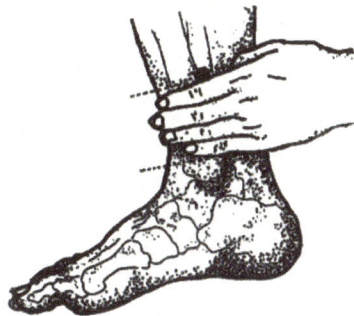

Move your thumb over the pressure point. You can let your other fingers gently wrap around your lower leg.

Press your thumb firmly into the pressure point. When you hit the point, it may feel sore.

Begin rubbing circles with your thumb until a contraction start. Stop rubbing during the contraction and rub again in between until the contractions become regular.

There are a few more acupressure points to induce labor which are less popular but you can try stimulating if the previous two points didn't bring on contractions.

GB21 (Jianjing) pressure point.

Draw an imaginary line between the prominent bone of the neck (C7), and the top of the shoulder joint. GB21 point lies midway along this curved line, at the highest point of the shoulder muscle. It feels tender when press and the sensation is stronger than any other points along this line. You can find this point on yourself by putting your hand on the shoulder and palpating with your index finger along this "imaginary line".

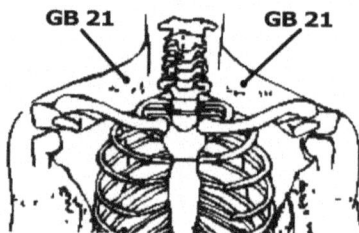

BL67 (Zhiyin) acupressure point.

This point lies on the little toe, just on the outside aspect of the toenail.

LIV3 (liver 3) acupressure point.

Located on the foot, just between the big toe and the second toe. Helps to relaxe and relieve the pain.

Note: Don't stimulate these acupressure points unless you are at least full term, or at 38 to 40 weeks gestation.

Chapter 4

Labour and Delivery

Childbirth is always a special and unique experience. No two deliveries are identical and there is no way to predict how your delivery is going to go. There's plenty you can do to prepare yourself, though. It helps if you know what to expect.

Childbirth usually occurs in three stages:

1st stage: From the beginning of true labour until the cervix is completely dilated to 10 cm.

2nd stage: The period after the cervix is dilated to 10 cm until the baby is delivered.

3rd stage: Delivery of the placenta.

1st stage of labour.

1st stage is the longest and also subdivided into three periods:

Early labour phase: The time from the beginning of labour until the cervix is dilated to 3 cm.

Active labour phase: The time when cervix dilates from 3 cm to 7 cm.

Transition phase: The time when cervix dilates from 7 cm to 10 cm (full dilation).

Early labour phase starts when your cervix starts to open and widen up to 3 cm. You may not notice this starting, as your uterus may be contracting very gently. You may even be several centimetres dilated before you realise you're in labour. Early labour will last approximately 8-12 hours.

What else can happen during this stage?

- You lose your mucous plug. Losing the plug is a sign of dilation and effacement of the cervix but the labour is still could be one or two days or even weeks away. Not everyone notices losing the plug. For some women it goes unnoticeable.
- You have a pink mucous discharge called "bloody show". Passing that bloody show means that the small blood vessels in the cervix are rupturing due to its dilation. This is a true sign that the labour is beginning and you'll have a baby soon (in a matter of hours or maybe even a day or two).
- The contractions become increasingly painful and that they're coming regularly. These are different to Braxton Hicks contractions, which are irregular and painless. Contractions will last about 30-45 seconds, giving you 5-30 minutes of rest between contractions.
- You can experience indigestion, diarrhoea, sensations of warmth in the abdomen.
- Your waters can break but it is more likely that they'll break during active labour.

What to do:

During this phase you should just try to relax. It is not necessary to rush to the hospital yet. Contractions usually start gradually, building up to a peak of intensity before fading away. You may have to stop and breathe through them. Relaxation techniques will help you to keep calm and control your breathing. Staying relaxed means your muscles are loose, making it easier for you to breathe more rhythmically. This allows you and your baby get more oxygen. So relaxation can help your baby to cope with labour, too.

Breathing relaxation or progressive muscle relaxation techniques would be helpful to use during this stage of labour.

- Try to rest or sleep during this stage preparing your body for active stage and delivery.
- During the day go for a walk or carry on with gentle activities.
- Eat light meals and drink plenty of fluid (don't eat anything heavy like burgers or potato chips). Foods to eat are: light soup or broth, toast, plain pasta or rice, pudding, jelly or a banana.
- Talk to a supportive friend or family member.
- Notify support people and check arrangements for childcare if you have other kids in the family.
- Time your contractions from the beginning of one to the beginning of the next.
- Remember to empty your bladder often. Full bladder can slow down the progress of labour.

For some women, early labour starts and stops. For others, it progresses into active labour. But don't worry, if the labour stops – it will start again. Your baby knows the right time to come out.

Active labour phase: your cervix will dilate 4-8 cm. This stage usually last about 3-5 hours.

- Contractions during this phase will last about 45-60 seconds with 3-5 minutes rest in between.
- Contractions become more painful.
- Back pain may continue to be a problem.
- You may have a show of blood and mucus or the membranes may rupture now or later in the first stage, if they haven't done so already.
- Leg discomfort increases.

Things you can do:

- Continue to drink plenty of fluid (water or juice).
- Suck on sweets to keep up your energy.
- Vary your position to keep as comfortable as possible (standing, kneeling, lying, down, straddling a chair, all fours).
- Have a bath or hot shower.
- Ask for a back rub or massage.
- Do whatever feels right - rock, sing, meditate, groan or even swear.
- Express your feelings as you wish. There's no right way to do this. Your needs may change as labour progresses.
- Continue with your relaxation techniques.

Real Fact: women who practice meditation and relaxation techniques during pregnancy experience much less pain, have less complications during labour and have a better chance to have a natural delivery.

Transition phase is when your cervix dilates from 8cm to 10cm. Transition will last about 30 min-2 hrs. Contractions during this phase will last about 60-90 seconds with a 30 second-2 minute rest in between. This is the hardest phase but also the shortest. Women feel this stage in different ways. It can be intense and overwhelming.

Contractions during this stage are 1 to 3 minutes apart, and lasting for approximately 50 - 70 seconds. Often there is no rest period in between.

You might experience hot flashes, chills, nausea, vomiting, or gas. Emotionally, you may feel vulnerable and overwhelmed, even discouraged, irritable or frustrated.

What you can do.

The best you can is to hang in there and remember that your baby is its way. To make the experience less painful you can:

- Ask for an epidural if the pain becomes very intensive.
- Ask to have a massage or a back rub if you think that touching might help you to ease the pain.
- Change your position. It can provide some relief – for example, if you're feeling a lot of pressure in your lower back, getting on all fours may reduce the discomfort. (see labour positions below).
- Ask for a cool cloth on your forehead or a cold pack on your back. It may feel good, or you may find a warm compress more comforting.

You may like to consider using natural pain relieve methods:

- As a way to distract you from the labour pain you can try to use some distractions like nice music or a pleasant conversation with a family member, friend or a birth coach.
- Try to visualize that those hard contractions are helping your baby make the journey out into the world. Try visualizing your baby moving down with each contraction.
- Doulas help. According to studies, women who use Doulas have 60% less requests for epidurals. A doula is a professional trained in childbirth who provides emotional, physical and informational support to the mother who is expecting, is experiencing labour, or has recently given birth. The doula's purpose is to help women have a safe, memorable and empowering birthing experience.
- Water immersion in labour can provide a lot of pain relief, relaxation and comfort for a labouring woman.
- You can use hypnosis and relaxation during birth.
- Homeopathic/Naturopathy remedies also can be a great help.

The good news is that if you've made it this far without medication, you can usually be coached through transition – one contraction at a time – with constant reminders that you're doing a great job and that the your baby's arrival is near.

2nd Stage of Labour: Pushing and Delivery.

Pushing and delivery of the baby can take anything from 20 minutes to 2 hours. Contractions become very strong and painful and last about 45-90 seconds at intervals of 3-5 minutes rest in between. Other things you can experience in the 2nd stage of labour:

- Strong natural urges to push.
- Tremendous rectal pressure.
- Baby's head will become visible.
- Can be a minor bowel or urination accident.
- Burning, stinging sensations during crowning.
- An increase in bloody show and slippery wet feelings as the baby emerges.

What you need to do when pushing:

- Get into a pushing position: semi-sitting or semi-squatting positions are often the best because you can use gravity to your advantage.
- When you feel the urge to push – you must push as much as you can.
- Relax your thighs, pelvic floor and anal area. If you have been doing Kegel exercises you know how to do that. Focus all your energy on your vagina and rectum and push as if you're having a big bowel movement. Do not strain your upper body or face: it can result in chest pain after delivery and blood shots on your eyes around them.
- Rest between contractions to help regain your strength.
- Don't get embarrassed if a bit of involuntary bowel move- ment or urine come out when you push. Nearly everyone

experience that during delivery. It happens because the rectum gets under tremendous pressure during delivery. Don't let embarrassment to interfere with the pushing rhythm.

- Use a mirror to view your progress. This can be very encouraging when you see your baby head crown. This gives you inspiration to push when your body feels weak and exhausted.
- Do not become discouraged if your baby's head emerges and then slips back into the vagina (this process can take two steps forward and one step back).
- Use your own breath to help you push. Take a few deep breaths while the contraction is building. At the peak of contraction take a deep breath and push when exhaling.

Labour positions.

There is no need to take labour lying down. The positions you decide to take will have an effect on your comfort level during contractions and your sense of control during contractions.

The positions you can adopt are many:

- Standing and leaning over something such as a bed or a chair.
- Standing and leaning back against something such as a wall.
- Sitting astride a chair, birth stool or fit ball and leaning forward onto the knees.
- Squatting.
- Going onto all fours and leaning over completely.
- Lying down flat on the back.
- Lying down on either the left or right side of the body.
- Sitting up with legs stretched out in front.
- Sitting in a legs crossed, somewhat elevated position.

3rd stage of labour. The third stage is the delivery of the placenta and it is the shortest stage. The time it takes to deliver your

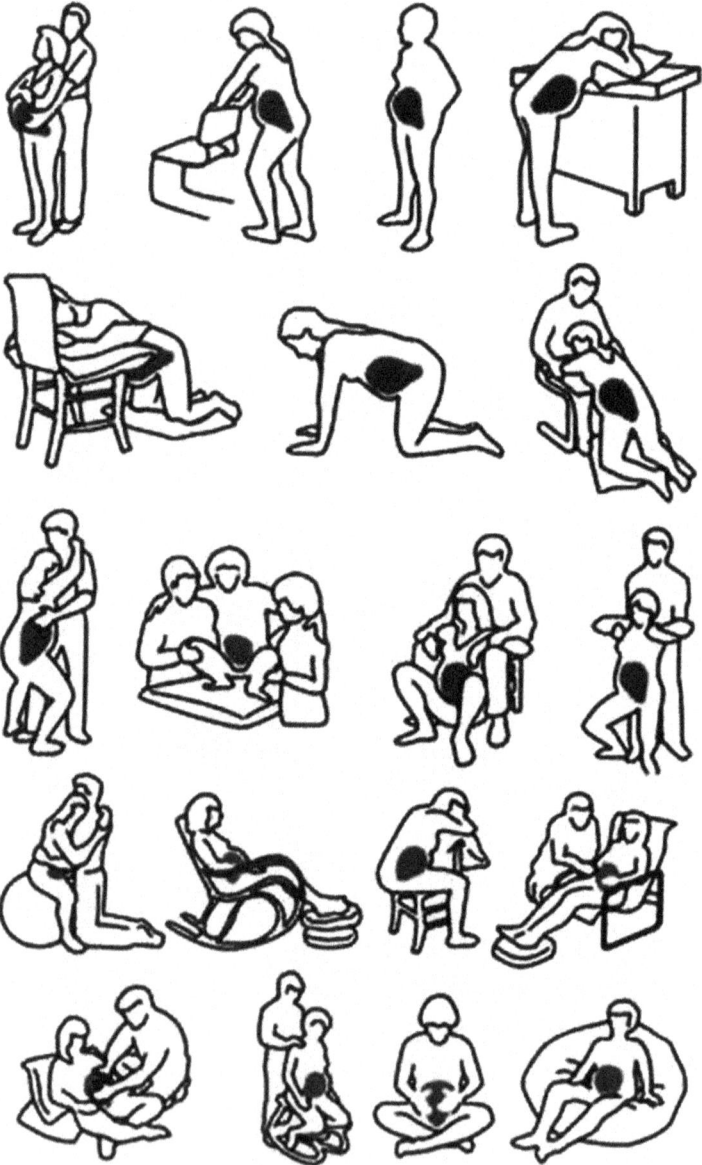

Labour positions

placenta can range from 5 to 30 minutes. Your practitioner will help deliver the placenta but before labour starts it is a good idea to consider whether to have an *actively managed or natural (physiological)* third stage.

What happens if you choose an actively managed third stage?

- An injection of oxytocin (which helps your uterus contract) is given into your thigh after the birth of your baby.
- You and your baby may be close and cuddling (skin to skin) and he/she may be nuzzling at the breast.
- The cord is clamped and cut (you may have delayed cord clamping if you wish).
- The midwife will check for evidence that the placenta has separated and then apply counter pressure above your pubic bone and deliver the placenta with gentle but firm traction on the cord. This process usually takes 5 to 10 minutes.
- If you have a water birth and choose to have active manage-ment, or your midwife recommends it, you will need to exit the pool for this stage of labour.

What happens if you choose a natural (physiological) third stage?

Following the birth of your baby:

- The cord is not clamped or cut and is left pulsating (provid-ing all is well with your baby).
- Your baby may be nuzzling at your breast.
- You will continue to feel mild to strong contractions at regu-lar intervals. The uteruspushes down with each contraction, leading to a gradual decrease in size. This helps the placenta separate from the wall of the uterus.
- You may feel a trickle of blood as the placenta separates from the wall of the uterus (this is normal).

- Being in an upright position will help you birth your placenta. Some women find it useful to position themselves on the toilet lined with a bowl to catch the placenta and any blood loss.
- If you have given birth to your baby in water and choose to birth your placenta naturally, you may remain in the pool, unless the midwife is concerned about your blood loss.
- As you feel a strong contraction and pressure in your bowel, you may feel an urge to push.
- Once the placenta has birthed the cord can be clamped and cut.
- This process can take from 10-60 minutes.

Can you change your mind about active vs. natural management of the 3rd stage?

Yes, you can change your mind about how you would like to birth your placenta at any time during your pregnancy or birth.

What kind of management is the safest?

Many clinical studies have shown that active management of placenta delivery is more effective than natural management in reducing the risk of heavy bleeding immediately after birth. For this reason, active management is considered the safest practice.

What you can do during the 3rd stage:

- Hold your new baby next to your skin and, if you're going to breastfeed, offer your breast as soon as possible. This will stimulate hormones to make the placenta separate faster.
- Help deliver the placenta by pushing if you're asked so. Your practitioner will let you know what to do.
- Hang in there during the stitching up any episiotomy or tears (you'll get a local anaesthetic for this).
- Be proud of your accomplishment!

Analgesia for childbirth.

You don't have to suffer the pain during childbirth. In fact, most women ask for pain relief during delivery. Several methods are available, including the use of drugs and nonpharmacological means. Pharmacological methods include Entonox (or gas and air), epidural, pethidine, spinal (local anaesthetic), morphine and others.

Non-pharmacological methods need to be taught during pregnancy by a trained person (antenatal classes are very helpful with that). Non-pharmacological methods include hypnosis, massage and touch, relaxation techniques, rhythmical movements, hot and cold showers or baths and transcutaneous electrical nerve stimulation (TENS). Some women find them very helpful in relieving pain during labour.

Hypnosis

Hypnosis for labour is hyper-focusing your attention away from the pain and altering your moods and sensations mentally. Hypnosis also helps to eliminate fears, allowing you to block out labour pain. Women can be coached to achieve the state of hypnosis during labour and follow their own suggestions for relieving pain. Most commonly used hypnotic suggestions are:

Transferring Numbness. Imagine that your hand is numb, as if placed in ice water. Then move the hand over the painful area to transfer the numbness there.

Time Distortion: View the time with pain as shorter and the time between painful episodes as lasting longer than in reality.

Imaginative Transformation: Interpret the pain as a benign, acceptable sensations (such as labour contractions being surges of energy that cause only a feeling of slight pressure) and, therefore, not problematic.

Hypnosis is a very safe option, and the fact that it does not require medication makes it a very attractive option for childbirth analgesia. But some women are not appropriate for hypnosis. Those, who are unable to follow verbal directions or have other medical illnesses, should not be offered hypnosis as a pain relieve during delivery. Other contra indications to hypnosis in labor are:

- Severe psychiatric illness such as paranoia or delusions.
- Severe mental retardation.
- Another medical illness presenting with pain.
- Active involvement in personal injury litigation related to pain.
- Little or no ability to be hypnotized due to disinterest or disbelief in its efficacy.
- Conflicts with religious beliefs.

Water Birth

Water birth is considered to be less painful. Contact with warm water relieve smuscles tension and reduces stress during labour.

Vocalization

You can relieve your labour pains by voicing your sensations. You can moan your contractions, softly sing, chant, or grunt. You should follow your body and know that whatever sounds you make are good and natural sounds.

Counter Pressure

Counter pressure is performed by applying pressure, usually significant pressure, to an area of discomfort. By using your hands and pushing, usually at or just above the sacrum, this will help put counter pressure where a woman is feeling the most pain. She may also tell you to move higher or lower, but the most frequent request is more pressure.

Hands and Knees position

This position is relatively easy to do and a great one for pain relief for some women. When she is on her hands and knees the baby is tipped slightly out of the pelvis giving it more room to rotate. Due to the decreased pressure on the cervix many women don't experience as much pain during the contractions. This position also allows for great counter pressure for the lower back.

Acupuncture and acupressure

Acupuncture, an ancient Chinese art, calms your body and reduces pain. Acupuncture requires a specialist to come and put needles in.

Acupressure is a simple, safe and effective technique that involves the manual stimulation of specific point on the body by applying pressure to them using the fingers, elbows, palms, or blunt-tipped instruments. Acupressure is easy and quick to learn. Anybody can do it. The most common acupressure points to relieve labour pains are:

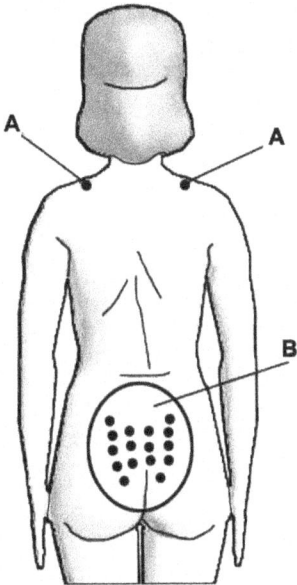

A –neck points;
B – buttock points

Neck points (A) the neck points can be found when the woman drops her head slightly forward, and a prominent bone can be felt or seen at the base of the neck (the 7th cervical bone). An imaginary curved line runs from the bony prominence of her neck, to the top of her shoulder joint. The points lie midway along this curved line, at the highest point of the shoulder muscle. The neck points should only be used in labour.

The buttock point (B) is a direct horizontal line from the top of the buttock crease. If you press along this line there will be a tender point

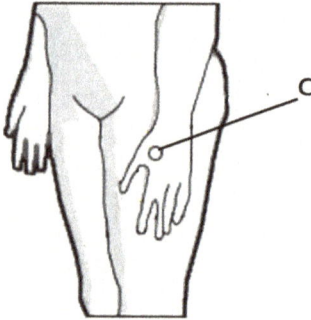

approximately two thirds of the distance between the buttock crease and the hipbone.

The hands points (C) in the webbing between the thumb and index finger at the highest spot of the muscle when the thumb and index finger are brought close together.

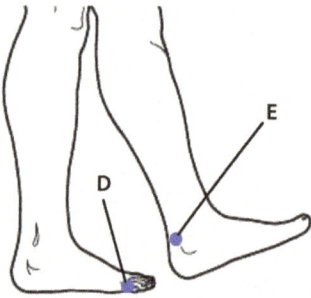

The little toe points (D) on the outside of the little toe, at the base of the toenail.

Achilles points (E) on each side of the Achilles tendon, located directly behind the ankle on the back of your foot, between the heel and the bottom of your calf.

Caution: do not stimulate Achilles points while pregnant, only for labour pains.

Deep Breathing

By focusing on your breathing patterns you can ease the pain of labour. Take a deep breath at the beginning of the contraction and, as you breathe out, re-lax. Then breathe in through your nose and breathe out through your mouth, keeping your mouth and cheeks very soft. Keep a good rhythm. Repeat this a few more times. Concentrate as hard as you can on breathing in as the contraction builds up, and out as it fades away.When the contraction is over, relax.

Caesarean Delivery

Statistic says that about 33%of all deliveries happen by caesarean section. You will not be able to participate actively at a caesarean delivery as you would at a vaginal delivery but, thanks to regional anaesthesia, most women are able to see and hear what is happening. Some caesareans are planned, some are emergency operations.

Sometimes there is a medical or obstetric reason to choose delivery via caesarean section long before the labour started. This is called planned caesarean. Emergency caesarean happens if a woman planed a vaginal birth but end up having an emergency caesarean birth, for medical or obstetric reasons.

There is a certain plan most caesarean birth follows:

1. **Preparation and anaesthesia:** begins with a routine IV during labour and anaesthesia — usually an epidural or spinal block, so the lower half of your body will be numb, but you'll remain awake. Your abdomen will be washed with antiseptic solution and the catheter will be inserted into your bladder. If you're having an emergency caesarean, there might not be time to numb you, in which case you'll given general anaesthesia for the duration of the section. You'll be sleeping during the delivery. When you wake up, expect to be groggy, disoriented, possibly sick to your stomach, and to have a sore throat from the endotracheal tube that was inserted to prevent any chance of your stomach contents coming back up during surgery and being inhaled, or aspirated, into your lungs.

2. **Incision:** after you get numb or asleep, a horizontal incision (just above your pubic hair line) will be made. Then the doctor makes another incision in the lower part of your uterus. One of two incisions is possible: a vertical cut down the middle of your uterus, or a low-transverse incision across the lower part of the uterus. Transverse incisions are used in 90% of caes are an these days because the muscle at the bottom of the uterus is thinner, so there will be less

bleeding (this type of cut is also less likely to split during subsequent vaginal deliveries).

3. **Getting the baby out:** after the amniotic fluid is suctioned out your baby will be brought into the world. The baby nose and mouth are suctioned and then you'll hear the cry. The umbilical cord will be quickly clumped and cut.

4. Placenta will be removed and the uterine incision will be repaired.

5. An injection of oxytocin will be given to you into your IV or intramuscularly to contract the uterus.

6. Antibiotics maybe given to minimise the chances of infection after the surgery.

Once your baby is born, you'll be moved to a post-op recovery room where you'll be closely monitored, usually for the next one to three hours. Your vital signs will be monitored carefully and the firmness of your uterus will be periodically checked. You'll see your baby soon after the C-section but the time depends on your condition.

Recovery tips:

- **Begin to move as quickly as you can.** Gentle exercises, such as light walking, can help a woman recover from a C-section faster.

- **Properly support the abdomen.** After having a C-section, things such as coughing or sneezing can be very painful. Supporting the abdomen with a small soft pillow can help reduce the pain, and reduce the risk of the incision reopening.

- **Keep the incision clean.** The incision should only be touched when the hands are clean, and at times of dressing changes. Strictly follow your doctor's recommendation regarding the stitches and incision.

- **Wear loose fitting and cotton clothing.** Loose fitting cotton clothing prevents the incision from becoming irritated and/or infected from clothing rubbing against it.
- Rest and use warm and cold compresses to the abdomen.
- Eat healthy and drink plenty of water.

Exercises after caesarean:

There are special exercises to help women regain strengthen in the muscles, ligaments and the whole body after caesarean:

1. Deliberately and loudly cough at least 10 times an hour, pulling your belly button into your spine. This exercise makes your abdomen stronger and promotes the healing of the wound.
2. Pull your belly to spine and squeeze your pelvic floor UP to your belly as you say "HUP HUPHUPHUPHUPHUP HUPHUPHUP" (10 HUPS) loudly and relax. Repeat several times a day.
3. Lying on your back (in bed), pull toes towards your body, then back. Repeat 10 times. Do 10 rotational movements clockwise, and then 10 rotational movement anticlockwise.
4. Lying on your back (in bed), tense your calf muscles and knees and relax. Repeat 10 times.
5. Lying on your back (in bed), tighten your buttocks and relax. Repeat 10 times.
6. Lying on your back (in bed), bend and stretch one leg, then the other. Repeat 10 times.

Self-Massage of the caesarean scar.

When your scar tissue is healing well (between 8-12 days after surgery) and your sutures or staples have dissolved or been removed, you can begin to do some gentle self- massage of the scar or hire an experienced postnatal massage therapist who can provide scar tissue massage. You should perform scar massage daily, at least twice a day for at least 10-15 minutes in the first three months. Your scar will start to flatten out instead of feeling like a raised bumpy line across your belly, and if performed successfully after several months you will no longer be able to feel your caesarean scar, you may only see it.

Massaging your caesarean scar for even a few minutes a day can have a huge benefit. In fact, knowledgeable self-massage is one of the best things you can do to avoid complications from adhesions and to improve the look and feel of your scar itself. Because massage helps to stimulate nerve endings, it can also be used to help relieve numbness and restore feeling where it has been lost.

Self-massage of the scar.

Start massage not earlier then 7-8 days after surgery. The scar should be well-healed and there are no signs of infection. It is always better to check with your doctor before you start the self-massage.

Make sure the scar is not sensitive to the touch, to help desensitize the area place a warm washcloth over scar and lightly rub with fingertips for 1-2 minutes. Once you are able to touch the scar without sensitivity or pain you are ready to massage.

Do the massage very gently without using a lot of pressure.

- First, test to see if any area of the scar feels stuck to underlying tissue, place your thumb and index finger on opposite ends of the scar and gently push your thumb and finger together. If your scar and skin make a rounded arch out away from your body, then outer layers of scar tissue are not adhered. If the scar looks more similar to an "M" with the center of the scar stuck and this forms an arch on either side, then you have scar tissue adhesions present. If you can't lift the scar away from your body you may have areas of tissue adhesion or you could still be a little swollen from the surgery.

- Next place your two index fingers upright to each other on the opposite sides of the scar and press gently down and towards each other. You do this as you move along the scar.
- Next place your fingers over the scar and gently move the scar in circles (clock-wise and counter clock-wise). Your fingers should not slide over the skin. This can help smooth out your scar. If one area feels more stuck than another, spend more time in the stuck area.
- Next lightly grasp one end of the scar between your thumb and index finger. Gently lift scar away from body, separating it from the underlying tissue. Gently move your fingers side to side for 30 seconds. Move your fingers to the center of the scar, repeat technique and then move to the opposite end of the scar, and repeat.

If after two to four weeks of massaging your scar, you still feel areas that seem stuck then you might want to see a healthcare professional.

CHAPTER 5

Self–Healing Exercises After Giving Birth

To maintain your health and wellbeing after giving birth it is important to start exercising as soon as you can after delivery. It is always safer to ask your doctor but generally you can start doing the following exercises on the second or third day after delivery if you had an uncomplicated birth. These exercises will help you to:

- Prevent thromboembolic complications.
- Prevent and treat constipation.
- Prevent and treat afterbirth urinary problems.
- Heal the genitals, abdomen and reproductive organs.
- Promote weight loss.
- Improve your cardiovascular fitness.
- Restore muscle strength.
- Boost your energy level.
- Improve your mood and relieve stress.
- Prevent and promote recovery from postpartum depression.

Postpartum exercises.

1. Lie on your back with both arms stretched a long your-sides. Relax. Move your arms out and up above your head and take a deep breath in. Then join your palms and bring them to your forehead. Then put your arms down along your sides and breathe out. Repeat 4-5 times. You can start doing this from the 2nd day after birth.

2. Lie on your back with both arms stretched along yoursides. Move your arms out (90 degrees angle with the body) and bend your torso to the left. Your left hand is sliding down your side and the right hand touches the head. Take a deep breath in when you bending. Then, straight your body and exhale. Do the same movement to the opposite side. Repeat 4-5 times to each sides. You can start doing it from the 2nd day after delivery.

3. Lie on your back with both arms stretched along your-sides. Bend your knees and pull your feet towards pelvis. Then, lift your bent legs above your abdomen pulling your knees towards your chest. Hold them for a few sec-onds. Then, put your feet down to the original position. Repeat the exercise 4-5 times. You can start on the third day after birth.

4. Lie on your back with both arms stretched along the sides. Bend your legs and put your feet firmly on the floor (or bed). Slowly lift your pelvis off the ground, resting on your head, shoulders and feet (take a deep breath in). Simulta-neously with the rise of the body, tighten your pelvic floor muscles (Kegels). Hold the position for a few seconds. Then relax and slowly put the body down on the floor (or bed). Exhale when lowering the body. Do this exercise 3-5 times from the 3rd day after birth.

For stronger women: when lifting the torso, do not hold the knees together, move them apart as much as you can.

5. Sit on the floor (or bed). Bend your body forward trying to touch your toes. First, you can do it bending your knee. Then you should try to reach your toes keeping the knees straight. Repeat 5 times starting from the 5th day after birth.

6. Lie on your back with both hands behind your head, your legs straighten. Pull your feet to the pelvis (inhale). Separate your knees and move them aside as much as you can (exhale). Put the knees together and straighten your legs (inhale). When pulling the legs, tighten your pelvic floor muscles (Kegels) and relax them when extending the legs. Repeat 2-3 times from the 4th day after birth. After the 5th day repeat 4-5 times.

7. Lie on your back with both arms stretched along yoursides. Pull your legs to the belly, alternately left and right (kind of walking in the air). Do this exercise for 10 seconds on the 4th day after delivery. After the 4th day do it for 20 sec.

For weaker women: you can imitate bike pedalling in the air instead of walking.

8. Lie on your on your stomach, put your head on your arms. Flex your knees and do circular movements with your feet. Start doing it from the 4th day after birth. Do it for 10-20 sec.

9. Lie on your on your stomach, legs extended, hands joined together, elbows separated to the sides, chin rests on the hands. Lift your head and upper body up (inhale) and gradually return to its original position (exhale). Repeat 2-3 times from the day 6th after birth.

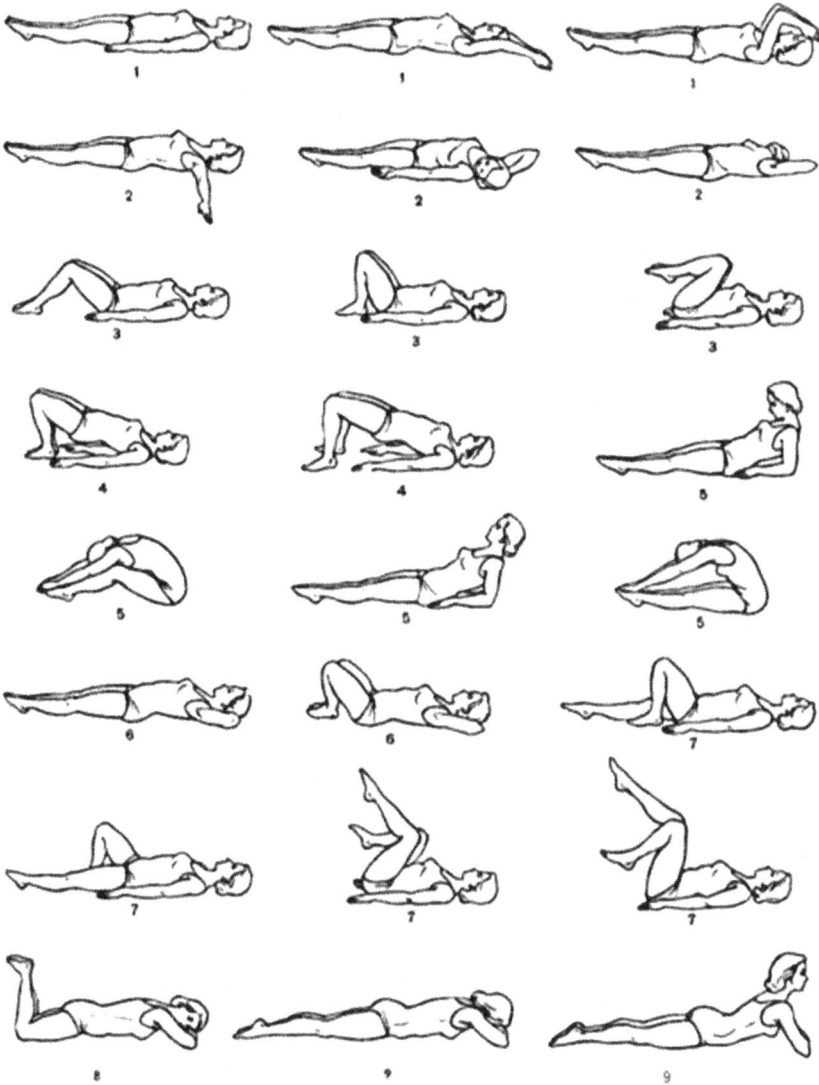

Postpartum exercises.

Post partum Self-massage.

One of the great ways to strengthen your abdominal muscles, improve your bowel activity and restore urination after birth is to do a self-massage of the abdomen with a tennis ball. You can do this self-massage on the second day after delivery if you have no birth complications.

How to do that?

- Empty your bladder before you start.
- Lie in bed and slightly bend your knees.
- Take a tennis ball, put it on your belly and put your hand on the ball.
- Start making circular motions (clockwise) from the navel and gradually increase the radius of movement until all the abdominal area is massaged.
- Press harder with every circle.
- Continue for 5-10 minutes.

This exercise should be done in the morning and then can be repeated 2-3 times a day, but not earlier than 2-3 hours after a meal.

CHAPTER 6

Stress and Tiredness during Pregnancy

Feeling tired and stressed is common during pregnancy. But too much stress can make you uncomfortable. To remain as stress-free as possible is certainly important during pregnancy as a stressed mother brings a stressed child; a loving mother brings a loving child.

The best way to keep stress at bay is thinking and feeling LOVE.

Accept all the changes of pregnancy with love and do everything you do - but with love. Of course, this is easier said than done, as pregnancy itself brings all sorts of feelings and mood swings. Then, love your feelings and mood swings too!!! Accept your feelings as an inevitable part of being pregnant and welcome them.

Many women find they're stressed and exhausted especially in the first trimester and then in the last trimester. This is your body's way of telling you that you need more rest, relaxation and self-love. After all, your body is working very hard to develop a whole new life.

Let's look at how stress can affect your pregnancy and the baby.

Excessive stress during pregnancy.

Excessive stress experienced by a woman during pregnancy may affect her unborn baby as early as 17 weeks after conception, with potentially harmful effects on brain and development.

Cortisol, which is pumped into the blood when you become anxious, is good in the short term, as it helps the body to deal with a stressful situation, but long-term stress can cause tiredness, depression and make you more prone to illness by supressing the immune system.

When you're pregnant, high level of stress can increase the chances of having a premature baby (born before 37 completed weeks of pregnancy) or a low-birthweight baby. Babies born too soon or too small are at increased risk for any sorts of health problems.

But not all stress is bad. The stress due to pregnancy discomforts is natural and normally harmless. Natural pregnancy stresses are:

- If you are dealing with the pregnancy symptoms such as nausea, constipation, being tired or having a backache.
- When your hormones are changing and cause your moods to change (mood swings due to pregnancy).
- You may be worried about what to expect during labour and birth or how to take care of your baby.
- If you worry about your job responsibilities while pregnant and how to prepare your employer for your maternity leave.
- Your life gets busy due to pregnancy and you feel a bit overwhelmed.

All these stresses (above) don't cause serious problems to your health or health of your baby, unless, of course you take it in a wrong way. A wrong way means not taking rest when it's needed, exacerbate the stress by focusing on negatives and talking yourself into more stress. A right way of stress handling means taking a lot of rest, making yourself relax, focusing on positive things, loving and accepting all the changes of life.

What types of stress can cause pregnancy problems?

Serious types of stress during pregnancy may increase your chances of certain problems. But don't' get discouraged, because most women who have serious stress during pregnancy can have healthy babies, especially if they have the right support and manage the stress well.

What kind of stress is considered to bea serious stress?

- Negative life events: divorce, serious illness or death in the family, or losing a job or home.
- Catastrophic events: earthquakes, hurricanes or terrorist attacks.
- Long-lasting stress: long-standing financial problems, being abused, having serious health problems or being depressed for a long time.
- Racism. Some women may face stress from racism during their lives.
- Underlying depression or anxiety disorders: some women may feel serious stress worrying about miscarriage, the health of their baby or about how they'll cope with labour and birth or becoming a parent. If you feel this way, talk to your doctor as soon as you can.

The effects of serious stress during pregnancy can be different: baby's growth restriction, decreased mother-baby bonding, preterm delivery and even miscarriages. Some studies have also shown that stress during pregnancy can increase risks for the children to have more allergies and schizophrenia.

Stress during pregnancy can often stop women to care for themselves which may mean not eating well or smoking and drinking alcohol. Stress also affects a woman's immune system and thus the baby's development.

Probably the most powerful antidote for all kinds of stress is positive *social support:* nurturing friends, kind words, and pleasant surroundings that prompt smiles and laughter are healing. Pregnant women who have this kind of support are less likely to react negatively to stress even to serious kinds of stress.

Pregnancy support groups can be a great help for women to get more social support. Talk to your health care provider about the availability of social support groups in your area.

Great stress antidotes during pregnancy.

Great stress antidotes are:

1. ***Regular exercise.*** Taking frequent effective exercise is one of the best physical stress-reduction techniques available. Exercise not only improves your health; it also relaxes tense muscles and helps you to sleep. Exercise essentially burns away the chemicals like cortisol and norepinephrine that cause stress. It pumps up your endorphins (pleasure hormones), improves your mood and makes you happy.

2. ***Meditation.*** It has been proven that meditation has many benefits on mental health: it heals depression, increases emotional positivity, and helps to deal with life's inevitable stresses.

   People often think of meditation as being nothing more than relaxation, but it's not true. Meditation and relaxation are not the same. Meditation involves relaxation (the cessation of unnecessary effort) but it also promotes mindfulness, which helps the stress-sufferer to recognize unhelpful patterns of thoughts that give rise to the stress response. Meditation also involves the active cultivation of positive mental states such as loving-kindness, compassion, patience, and energy.

3. *Relaxation techniques.* Many people associate relaxation with zoning out in front of the TV at the end of a stressful day. But this does little to reduce the damaging effects of stress. To effectively combat stress, we need to activate the body's *natural relaxation response.* You can do this by practicing relaxation techniques such as deep breathing, meditation, rhythmic exercise, and yoga. These activities, if done correctly, produce natural relaxation response in your body, reduce everyday stress and boost your energy and moods. Several positive changes occur in the body and brain when you start practicing relaxation techniques regularly:

    - Slowing your heart rate
    - Lowering blood pressure
    - Slowing your breathing rate
    - Increasing blood flow to major muscles
    - Reducing muscle tension and chronic pain
    - Improving concentration
    - Reducing anger and frustration
    - Boosting confidence to handle problems

4. *Eat Healthy.* Eating wrong food makes you vulnerable to everyday stress. Bad food is a stress factor on its own because it is difficult for the body to digest it. In addition, bad food leaves too many toxins in the body which can make you stressed out even more. Bad foods are: all fatty foods, sugary foods and processed foods. Eating more fresh vegetables and fruits, fish and lean meat, low fat dairy products is beneficial for stress reduction and making you healthier.

5. *Find a hobby.* Doing something for the fun of it is a great way to relive stress. While there are many great hobbies to choose from, this is a list of hobbies that are particularly useful in relieving stress: needlepoint, bird watching, gardening, explore photography, scrap booking, maintaining an aquarium, puzzles, drawing, painting, knitting, playing the piano and writing.

6. *Get a regular whole body massage.* Massage therapy is one of the best antidotes for stress. If even the untrained hands of a friend or partner can soothe aches and pains, and diminish anxiety, then imagine the effect of a therapeutic massage by a trained practitioner.

7. *Self-massage.* You can massage many parts of your body yourself. These body parts are: face and head, legs and feet, arms and hands, shoulders and neck. Self-massage is a great way to heal muscle knots or "trigger points" which are small patches of super-contracted muscle fibres that cause aching and stiffness. They can affect performance of the whole muscle, spread pain and cause lots of stress. You can often get even more relief from self-massage than you can get from a massage therapist. Professional help is nice, but it can also be expensive and time consuming. So, self-massage is a safe, cheap, and reasonable approach to self-help for stress and common pain.

8. *Acupuncture.* The purpose of acupuncture is to unblock a person's energy pathways or "qi". According to Chinese medicine blocking of energy pathways or "qi" is the cause of stress and other illnesses.

9. *Foot rubs (or foot massage).* Have your husband (or other relative or even a friend) give you one. You can also massage your feet yourself. Massaging the feet can alleviate anxiety and bring about a deep state of relaxation. One

important point that is situated on both feet is the solar plexus reflex. When the solar plexus point is pressed on, stress is released and the body is renewed. To find the solar plexus point draw an imaginary line from the point between you fourth and fifth toes to the highest point of your arch. Identify the general location of the solar plexus zone as the midpoint of this line. You will know that you have found the solar plexus zone when you feel a pinpoint of pain. Apply firm pressure to this point for 20 to 60 seconds and release. Repeat this several times on both feet to relieve tension.

10. **Get regular orgasms** (unless contra indicated in pregnancy). Sexual activity and orgasm are shown to reduce stress due to the surge of oxytocin, the so-called "cuddle hormone," that occurs with orgasm. What's more, studies show that orgasms regulate blood pressure level which is also important especially when pregnant. Orgasms help you sleep better. In addition to increasing trust, attachment and bonding, the post-orgasm hormone oxytocin triggers a cascade of bodily events, including the release of other feel-good hormones called endorphins. These endorphins often have a sedative effect and also make you happy.

11. **Write a daily journal.** By writing your emotions and your feelings about things, you become more aware of yourself and how you respond to your environment. You are then better able to handle situations. You are more likely to stop and think about the problem and try to resolve it rather than be overwhelmed by it.

12. **Take regular naps.** You can get incredible benefits from 15 to 20 minutes of napping. You reset the system and get a burst of alertness and increased attention. It also reduces stress and makes you calm and relaxed.

13. **Yoga.** Yoga can improve depressive symptoms and immune functions, as well as decrease chronic pain, reduce stress, and lower blood pressure. Yoga, which derives its name from the word, "yoke"—to bring together—does just that, bringing together the mind, body and spirit.

Managing stress and the level of tiredness is all about making lifestyle and work changes. Try not to be so controlling about your life and 'let it go' more often. Allocate the work to other people and accept their help. Just think that your main job now is to carry a healthy child and this is your first responsibility.

So, read, talk to friends, talk to your husband, take walks, swim and enjoy life as much as possible. If all is not enough get professional help.

Practical techniques to manage stress and exhaustion during pregnancy.

1. Learn to centre yourself. "Centering" is simply returning all of your scattered energies to the centre of yourself. That allows you to focus on the present moment without worrying and thinking of the past or future. It makes you to become whole and aware, especially in times of stress or worry, when the mind can become easily distracted.

Meditation to centre yourself while pregnant.

Sit comfortably on the floor in a quiet place, cross-legged. You can also sit on a chair – whatever you like the best. Close your eyes. Adjust your position so that you are balanced and keep your back as straight as possible. Put your hands on your lap. Take in a deep breath and let it out completely. Imagine yourself inhaling white cleansing energy and exhaling dark, dusty 'busy-ness' and futile wheel-spinning. This process can take 10-15 minutes while you're first learning it, but once you learn the 'centered' feeling, you can center yourself with a few breaths at any time, even while talking to people, driving your car or walking into that important meeting.

People have different concepts of where their center is. Some people feel that their center is behind their bellybutton. Some people locate it at their heart chakra or their solar plexus chakra. The important thing is to pull your energies into a tight ball at the location where you feel your center is and focus on this center instead of having scattered attention.

Why centering is important?

Centering eliminate stress, put all your attention inside yourself, make you become neutral which is the most natural and healing state.

2. **Ground yourself**. Grounding connects you to the energy of the earth. It is important in healing and stress relieve since it prevents you from depleting your own body's energy. Simply put, you connect to the earth by imagining you are connected to the earth. Sounds silly, but it works. Here's how you do it:

Meditation to ground yourself while pregnant.

Imagine you are standing in your bare feet on the ground. (It doesn't matter where you actually are). Your feet are planted firmly on the bare earth, and by an exercise of your will, you send roots into the earth. As you inhale, you draw energy up through your new 'roots', and as you exhale, you send your roots even further into the earth. Do this for several minutes - you should definitely feel a change in the state of your feeling of 'aliveness'.

Grounding brings you calmness, stamina and put your body into a healing state.

3. **Shield yourself.** Shielding is the process of protecting yourself from the energetic influences around you. You can create your own special shielding ritual but here is the basic technique you can use.

Meditation to shield yourself while pregnant.

First, center yourself by invoking feelings of love then imagine a white protective light of energy like a cocoon enveloping around you. This will act like a protective energy around you, it is important to focus on the intention that no negative energy can penetrate this shield to affect you.

When making your shield, associate some trigger word to your meditation so that when you are around others and feeling affected by their negative energy, you can quickly get into the mind set with the trigger word you have chosen. Then use this trigger word every time you reinforce your energy shield, so that it will become automatically associated and familiar in your mind. This will enable you to raise your protective shield at any time you are feeling drained by the negative energies of other people.

4. **Use mantra** whenever you need to redirect your thoughts and stop thinking negatively. Mantra is a word or phrase that you repeat to yourself again and again for a specific effect. It works on your subconscious mind (where emotions come from).
   - I love myself
   - I am free from anger
   - I am free from sadness
   - Love is my experience

It can be just "Ommmmm...." repeated on each long exhale or any other bodily sound that you think can please your body. According to Hinduism, OM is the primordial sound from which all creation arose.

Om Namah Shivaya – sanskrit for: "I honour the God within."

The main point in using mantras is not to intellectualize it. Just focus on the sound or your body vibrations during the sound, that's it. Fully accept it as helpful, no questions, no concerns and no thoughts. Just be.

How to do it?

Mantra Meditation.

Just sit comfortably, close your eyes, take a deep breath to relax and start slowly repeating one of the mantras. Focus on its sound, don't dwell on meaning. Repeat it again and again.

If none of the mantras above meet your needs, you may develop your own mantra. Remember that it has to be short and easy to remember, it has to be positive and it has to have meaning for you.

5. **Use positive affirmations.** Affirmations are sentences with positive meanings which have to be repeated aloud. Affirmations are good for changing the meaning of your thoughts and eventually they can change a whole mindset. Examples:
   - Pregnancy is safe for me and my baby
   - My baby loves me
   - I am a strong woman
   - I am a good mother
   - Everything is fine and I am completely relaxed

Read the chapter 'Positive Affirmations for Pregnancy' for more information on how to do affirmations during pregnancy.

6. **Get at least eight hours of sleep every night**, and a nap during the day when possible. Start sleeping on your left side. This will relieve pressure on major blood vessels that supply oxygen and nutrients to the fetus. If you have high

blood pressure during pregnancy, it is even more important to be on your left side when you are lying down.

7. **Meditate daily.** For the best result you can start and finish your day with a 20 minutes meditation. During the day take short breaks from what you do and meditate 5-10 min. Read 'meditation during pregnancy' chapter.

8. **Join pregnancy-yoga classes or do it at home on your own.** Yoga poses help to relieve discomfort and release tension in your body. Read 'The Yoga for Pregnancy' chapter.

9. **Use Natural Smells and Aromatherapy**. There are some plans and natural products which smell can make you happier, more relaxed and even induce the production of pleasure chemicals in the body. These smells are:
   - Smell of freshly baked bread
   - Peppermint (boost moods and motivation)
   - Apples smell
   - Lavender
   - Fresh Coffee smell or coffee beans smell

These smells are definitely safe and can make a big difference in how you feel during pregnancy. Smell them and feel the difference.

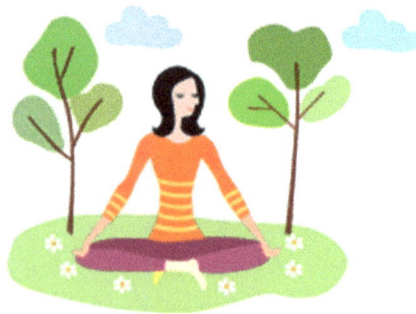

CHAPTER 7

Morning Sickness

More than half of all pregnant women experience discomfort from the nausea and vomiting associated with pregnancy, so you are definitely not alone in this journey you are traveling.

What is the reason for morning sickness?

Unfortunately, no one is exactly sure what causes morning sickness. The cause seems to be a combination of issues related to:

- High levels of hormones, including oestrogen
- Fluctuations in blood pressure, particularly lowered blood pressure
- Altered metabolism of carbohydrates
- The interplay of enormous physical and chemical changes that pregnancy triggers.
- An enhanced sense of smell
- Excess stomach acids
- Stress and fatigue that commonly accompany pregnancy.

How to Cope up with Morning Sickness?

- Don't take drugs of any kind, unless your doctor knows you are pregnant and has prescribed specific medications.

- Eat a few dry crackers before getting out of bed in the morning.
- Ginger: use in the form of cookies to 2 - 3 pieces before you get up in the morning, in the form of tea (freshly ground ginger, brewed with hot water), the juice (a slice of ginger and apple mix with a mixer).
- Avoid low blood sugar: Eat a small amount of snacks at regular intervals.
- Learn acupressure points.
- Put a small amount of peppermint oil on a sugar cube and slowly suck it.
- Add cardamom powder to yoghurt and other foods.
- Don't try to eat anything that you suspect will make you nauseous.
- Eat small meals regularly, since an empty stomach tends to trigger nausea.
- Limit or eliminate fatty and spicy foods.
- Choose high carbohydrate and high protein foods.
- Avoid cooking or preparing foods whenever possible.
- Drink plenty of fluids, preferably water (add a sprig of fresh Mint and a slice of Ginger)
- Vitamin B6 supplements can be useful, but doses above 200mg per day can actually be harmful.
- Wear loose clothes that don't constrict the abdomen.
- Suck on ice if the nausea if acute.

Herbal remedies for Morning Sickness

Ginger: Ginger tea helps to stop nausea in many women. To make it, steep 2 teaspoon grated ginger in 2 cups of boiling water for 10 min, then let it cool to room temperature and sip it throughout the day. Do not prepare a stronger tea or drink more than 2 cups a day.

Dandelion: Dandelion tea also can help to stop nausea. Put 2 tablespoons of dried dandelion root in 2 cups of boiling water and steep it for 4 hours. Let it cool and drink slowly throughout the day. Do not drink more than two cups a day.

Cardamom: Cardamom can be drunk as a tea as well, and can also be added to the tea with the ginger. It should be prepared by placing four cardamom pods and three cups of water in a pot, and heated until small bubbles begin to appear. Do not boil it. Remove the pan from the heat and allow it to sit for 30 minutes. Strain and drink it. You can add on honey, if you like it sweet.

Mint: The anaesthetic constituents in mint work to minimize nausea by reducing the stomach's gag reflex. Make a cup of mint tea any time you feel a wave of nausea about to come. Place 1 tablespoon mint leaves in a 2 cups of boiling water. Let stand 20 to 30 minutes, shaking occasionally. Strain and sip as needed.

Fennel: Fennel seed is a nausea remedy from Chinese folk medicine. As with mint, fennel seed contains anesthetic constituents that may reduce queasiness. Crush 1 tablespoon fennel seeds into a coffee grinder. Place the crushed seeds in a cup and fill with boiling water. Cover and let steep for ten minutes. Drink the tea in sips to treat nausea.

Alfalfa: Alfalfa is usually used in form of tablets. You should follow the direction on the packet according to the tablets strengths.

Chamomile: Chamomile tea can help to relieve morning sickness.

Some certain smells can help to relieve morning sickness. These smells are: lavender, thyme, lemon, dill, fresh ginger and peppermint.

Homeopathy for morning sickness.

You may like to try homeopathic remedies to relieve the symptoms of nausea and vomiting. It is always the best to talk to a qualified homeopath about the prescription to suit your precise symptoms. But you can start from the following homeopathic remedies (below) and see a homeopath if your symptoms do not improve after five days.

Homeopathic remedies.	Your symptoms.
Recommendation: Choose the 30c strength of tablet	
Nux vomica	You have bitter or sour reflux, a metallic taste in your mouth; feel bloated, irritable and worse if you wear tight clothing.
Pulsatilla	Your reflux tastes of food you have recently eaten and your stomach feels empty and gurgles a lot. Also if you feel worse in the evenings and after eating fatty food, or are emotional and tearful, with changeable moods.
Natrummur	You have watery sweet reflux, cramping abdominal pressure, feel worse after eating starchy foods, and keep your emotions to yourself.
Dausticum	You have greasy, fatty-tasting reflux; feel over-full, feel worse if you are wet or cold, and feel hopeless about your condition.

Acupressure for morning sickness.

From a Chinese medicine perspective, energy channels called meridians make up the anatomy of human body. Acupressure points are points that lie on these energy channels (meridians). Morning sickness or nausea is seen as Qi (energy) going in the wrong direction. Your stomach energy should go down and out;

Acupressure points for morning sickness

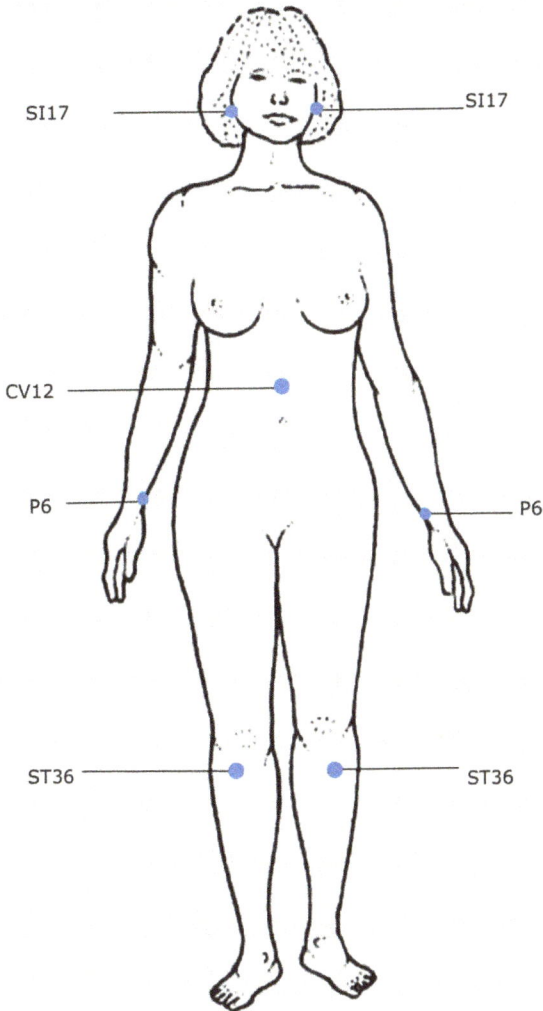

not up. By using the following acupressure techniques, you can help to restore the correct direction of energy flow.

Acupressure point P6. This is the most important point to use for nausea. It's located three finger-widths (or two thumbs) from your wrist on your forearm. Take a look at the inside of your left wrist crease. Use your thumb to measure 2 thumb widths back towards your elbow crease. This point is called "Pericardium six" because it lies on the Pericardium meridian. It has a connection to the inner lining of your stomach and has the effect of calming your mind. Start pressing deeply between the two tendons you can see there. If you can't see the tendons, bend your hand towards your elbow crease and claw your fingers, this will bring the tendons up for you to see. You will also notice that the two bones of your arm come together here at your wrist. This is the place you start to press – at the join of the bones in between the tendons. Press deeply – if it hurts in a "good" way, you are on the right spot – if not, move a little more towards your elbow crease and try again. Keep moving around this spot until you find some relief.

Acupressure point ST36. To find this point, place your fingers just outside your shin bone on the front of your lower leg. Move your big toe, and you will feel movement in the area of the point. Press in this area about four finger-widths below your kneecap.

Acupressure point SI17 is a point just under your earlobe where your jaw bone begins. It may be tender, but press as firmly as it is comfortable for several minutes.

Acupressure point CV12 is located in the middle of the abdomen and is used to treat heartburn, nausea, and poor digestion.

Before you start self-treatment, make sure that you're not dehydrated from vomiting. Signs of dehydration are: increased thirst, dry mouth and swollen tongue, weakness, dizziness, palpitations (feeling that the heart is jumping or pounding), confusion (a sign of serious dehydration), sluggishness, fainting, inability to sweat, decreased urine output. Dehydration is dangerous for you and your baby. If you have dehydration symptoms, first of all you'll need to restore your body hydration. Drink plenty of fluids and call your doctor.

Severe vomiting - Hyperemesis gravidarum.

For some women, the nausea of the first trimester is so severe that they become malnourished and dehydrated. These women may have a condition called 'hyperemesis gravidarum' (HG). HG refers to women who are constantly nauseated and/or vomit several times every day for the first 3 or 4 months of pregnancy.

You have higher risk of developing HG if:

- You're pregnant with twins or triplets.
- Family history of HG (your sister or mother had it).
- You had HG during your past pregnancy.
- You're prone to travel sickness or migraines.
- You have a pre-existing liver disease.

HG keeps pregnant women from drinking enough fluids and eating enough food to stay healthy. Many women with HG lose more than 5% of their pre-pregnancy weight, have nutritional problems, and may have problems with the balance of electrolytes in their bodies. Many women with HG have to be hospitalized so they can be fed fluids and nutrients through a tube directly into their veins. Usually, women with HG begin to feel better by the 20th week of pregnancy. But, some women vomit and feel nauseated throughout all three trimesters.

If you think you might be vomiting excessively, call your doctor.

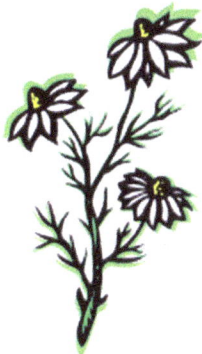

Chapter 8

What to Avoid during pregnancy

When you're pregnant you need to watch what you eat, what environment you are in and what you're doing. You don't want to be exposed to any harm while you are pregnant.

Some foods, some environments and some exercises (or activities) are not recommended during pregnancy.

Let's look at them all, starting from what *foods to avoid*.

Avoid Eating Fish that have high Mercury Levels: When you're fishing for dinner, steer clear of shark, swordfish, king mackerel, fresh tuna, tilefish, mahimahi, grouper, and amberjack. And limit your consumption to 340 g a week of shellfish, smaller ocean fish, farm-raised fish, canned light tuna, and freshwater fish. Limit canned albacore to 170 g per week.

Raw fish and seafood: Raw fish and seafood can contain bacteria and parasites which are dangerous for your health and especially your baby's health. Don't eat sushi that contains raw fish. Always cook fish until it flakes; shellfish must be firm. Stay away from uncooked marinated seafood — no amount of citrus juice or hot sauce is capable of killing dangerous bacteria. Also, cold smoked fish should stay off the menu because of the danger of Listeria (it's okay if cooked, as in a casserole).

Undercooked or raw meat and poultry: uncooked meat and poultry can contain lots of bacteria and parasites, such as E. coli, Trichinella, and Toxoplasma which are extremely dangerous for the baby. Always cook meat and poultry until they're well done.

Soft cheeses: Sometimes, soft cheeses contain Listeria, which is bacteria that can easily be passed on to your baby and cause many health problems including stillbirth and premature labour. Babies born to infected mothers can develop serious problems such as: meningitis, pneumonia, thrombocytopenia, anaemia, and sometimes conjunctivitis.

Stay away from soft cheeses including queso fresco, Brie, Camembert, feta, goat cheese, or Roquefort. Any pasteurized soft cheeses are fine, but if you're desperate for a chunk of Brie, make sure it's domestic and pasteurized — or cook it until it's bubbling before you dig in (for the same Listeria reason, heat cold cuts until steaming before serving, too).

Raw eggs: Raw eggs often contain Salmonella which is a dangerous bug. Also look out for raw eggs in homemade ice cream, cookie dough, mayonnaise, and eggnog, which often contain raw eggs.

Avoid alcohol: Drinking alcoholic beverages during pregnancy can have serious consequences for your baby, including birth defects and complications. Even moderate drinking can cause problems, so it's best to abstain entirely until after delivery. (Don't worry, however, if you had a couple of drinks before you found out you were pregnant.)

Avoid food-borne infections: Use the highest standards of hygiene when eating, cooking, handling and cleaning food!

Food-borne illness can cause serious health problems for both mother and baby.

Environmental hazards to avoid.

Avoid chemicals. Products that contain herbicides, pesticides, paint, stains, and some cleaning solutions may be harmful to your baby. If you must use these things, wear gloves, a mask and keep the room well-ventilated.

Avoid cleaning or changing a cat's litter box. This could put you at risk for an infection called 'toxoplasmosis'. Toxoplasmosis is caused by a parasite that cats can carry in their faces. Toxoplasmosis is dangerous for a baby.

Avoid taking very hot baths, hot tubs, or saunas. High temperatures can be harmful to the foetus or cause you to faint.

Avoid using scented feminine hygiene products. Pregnant women should avoid scented sprays, sanitary napkins and bubble bath. These products might irritate your vaginal area, and increase your risk of a urinary tract infection or yeast infection.

Avoid using a douche. Douching can irritate the vagina, force air into the birth canal and increase the risk of infection.

Avoid having optional x-rays. X-rays are a form of radiation that may be linked to a very small risk of cancer for an unborn baby. But x-rays are usually safe during pregnancy. If your doctor says you need x-rays for a health problem. you should follow their advice. But, sometimes doctors can use other tests in place of x-rays. At other times, x-rays can wait until after the baby is born.

Avoid smoking tobacco. Tell your doctor if you smoke. Quitting is hard, but you can do it. Ask your doctor for help. Smoking during pregnancy passes nicotine and cancer-causing drugs to your baby. Smoke also keeps your baby from getting needed nourishment and raises the risk of stillbirth and premature birth (a small baby born early).

Avoid drinking alcohol. Stop drinking alcohol.

Don't use illegal drugs. Tell your doctor if you are using drugs. Marijuana, cocaine, heroin, speed (amphetamines), barbiturates and LSD are very dangerous for you and your baby.

All medications should be avoided during that vital first three months unless prescribed by your doctor who knows you are pregnant.

Activities to avoid during pregnancy.

As your pregnancy progresses, you should avoid any activities that put you at risk for falling or increase the chance of trauma to your abdomen. The following activities can cause problems during pregnancy and generally should be avoided:

- Contact sports: Soccer, basketball, and hockey put you at a high risk of injury from a ball or puck, a collision with another player, or a fall during play.
- Downhill skiing should be avoided because of the risk of serious injuries and hard falls.
- Cycling isn't a good idea for newbies, but experienced riders may be able to continue until their second trimester. After the 3rd month of pregnancy cycling should be stopped. A shifting centre of gravity affects balance when the pregnancy progresses; this can cause falls and makes cycling dangerous.
- Gymnastics: it brings unnecessary risk of falling and increased chance of trauma to your abdomen.
- Horseback riding: Even if you're a good rider, it's not worth risking a fall.

- Tennis: This is okay in the 1st trimester if you're an experienced player. But you should stop it in the second and third trimester.
- Amusement park rides: Water slides and other rides at amusement parks should be avoided, since a forceful landing or sudden start or stop could harm your baby.
- Post-sport tubs and saunas: Soaking in hot tubs and Jacuzzis or sitting in a sauna can be dangerous to your developing baby because overheating has been linked to birth defects.

Absolute 'no-no' is for activities like scuba diving, snowboarding, surfing and water-skiing.

CHAPTER 9

Herbal Remedies during Pregnancy

There are many herbs that can help to heal almost any aches or complaints during pregnancy. You have to be aware though that not every herb or plant can be completely safe during pregnancy. Herbs may contain substances that can cause miscarriage, premature birth, uterine contractions, or injury to the foetus. Still not enough research has been done to measure the effects of various herbs on pregnant women or a developing foetus.

Here we discuss the herbs what have been traditionally used for different pregnancy complaints. These herbs have been proven to be safe during pregnancy. But every person is different, so before you take any herbs, please ask your doctor about its individual safety for you.

1. Increasing your Fertility.

   Using certain healing herbs can help to increase your fertility and your chances of conceiving. There are many herbs to help you with that. To choose the right herbs you need to know what is yourproblem regarding fertility. It can be irregular menstrual cycle, stress, decreased libido or any other problems related to body organs and systems.

Herbs which encourage pregnancy are characterized by their ability to:
- Nourish the uterus and especially the inner lining where implantation occurs.
- Nourish the entire body.
- Relax the nervous system and eliminate stress.
- Improve and balance normal hormonal function.
- Improve and balance sexual desire.

Here are the most commonly used herbs that can increase your change of conceiving a baby.

- **Vitex** is one of the most used herbs for boosting fertility in women as it regulates the hormones. It helps regulate irregular menstrual cycles and heavy bleeding.

- **Red Raspberryleaf** is an excellent source of calcium, magnesium and iron. It helps strengthen the uterine lining and lengthens the luteal phase of a menstrual cycle, enhancing the possibility of implantation.

- **Nettles** is high in calcium and iron content, nettles are extremely nourishing to the reproductive and adrenal systems. It improves hormonal balance. In combination with red clover and peppermint it can be a great tea to drink and a very good fertility booster.

- **Oatstraw** is a mild nourishing tonic herb. It is a mild aphrodisiac and also a wonderful hormone balancer.

- **Damiana** is a wonderful aphrodisiac and helps promote fertility in men and women. It can help balance irregular menstrual cycles and helps nourish the reproductive system.

- **Maca** is a root native to Peru. It is taken dried in capsule form. It helps increase sperm count and is great for boosting the libido in both men and women.

- **Alfalfa** is a great tonic herb; it is a phytoestrogen, which would be helpful when oestrogen is fluctuating (like it does in menopause). It also helps nourish the reproductive organs in both men and women. It is vitamin rich and will keep you healthy.

- **Red clover** is an all-purpose fertility booster. It is also a blood purifier. This herb takes a while to build up in the system though so it is best to start taking it a few months before trying to conceive.

- **False Unicorn** has been used in Native American healing for centuries to promote fertility. False Unicorn helps with male impotence as well as promoting a healthy menstrual cycle as well as recurrent miscarriages.

- **Saw Palmetto** is a great fertility herb for men it helps nourish the reproductive system and promote fertility. It can also be used my women for regulating your cycle.

2. **Herbs to use when you got pregnant.**
   Many herbs can be used to cope with different complaints of pregnancy. To make your experience safe, always ask your practitioner about using each herb in a particular situation.

   Herbs for reliving morning sickness:
   - Chamomile tea: drink it as soon as you get up in the morning.
   - Ginger tea helps for morning sickness and can be used as a general tonic. You can make a hot ginger tea or add it to food. To make ginger tea: steep 1 teaspoon of freshly grated ginger in 1 cup of boiling water for 10 min, let it cool to room temperature, and sip it throughout the day.

- Dandelion sweetens the sour feeling, calms and strengthens the stomach, and improves the appetite.
- Peppermint oil aroma relieves nausea. Fill a large bowl with hot water. Place two drops of peppermint essential oil in the bowl and place it on a table near your bed.

Herbs for Soothing Indigestion and Heartburn.
- *Almonds.* A natural chemical in raw almonds helps tone the sphincter between the oesophagus and stomachso that acid stays in the stomach so you don't experience heartburn.
- *Meadowsweet* is one of the best digestive herbs for pregnant women. To make meadowsweet tea: put a tablespoon of the herb in a cup, pour 1 cup of boiling water over it, steep for 20 min, strain and drink. Drink three to four cups a day by sipping each cup slowly.
- Other herbs that can help with indigestion and heartburn are: Slippery elm, Fennel seed tea, Ginger tea, chewing a few basil leaves, chamomile tea.

Herbs for Increasing Tonus and Relieving Stress.
- Oats is high in calcium and magnesium; it builds healthy bones and nourishes the nervous system. This is the perfect herb to relieve nervous exhaustion and improve sleep. It is also high in fibre content, so can be good to relieve constipation during pregnancy. Can be taken as oatmeal cereal in the morning, along with oatmeal bread. Oatstraw tea has a mild flavour that can be used alone or mixed with other herbs. And a warm oatmeal bath is not only relaxing; it softens skin and relieves the itch of a growing belly.
- Nettle can also be used in the 1st trimester as it is a storehouse of nutrition (high iron and calcium content, as well

as an excellent source of folic acid). Nettle strengthens the kidneys and adrenals and relieves fluid retention. Nettle also strengthens veins and can prevent varicose veins and hemorrhoids. Nettle tea has a rich, green taste and can be mixed with other herbs. Cooked nettle is a mineral rich substitute for spinach and an excellent side dish with a dash of lemon juice and sesame seeds.

- Rose petals is a lovely herb for balancing the mood and increasing tonus. Traditionally used as a blood tonic.

Herbs for easing constipation:

First of all eat lots of fruits and vegetables especially plums, apples, figs, beetroot and cabbage.

Senna can help treat pregnancy constipation. A plant found in supplements and tea, senna contains anthraquinones (compounds that act as powerful laxatives). Side effects of senna are cramping and nausea. It should be avoided by people with heart conditions and digestive disorders (including ulcerative colitis and Crohn's disease). Talk to your doctor before using senna for pregnancy constipation.

Other herbs can be used for constipation during pregnancy are cascara sagrada, rhubarb and aloe. They should be used with care as they have certain side effects. Ask your practitioner about their safety for you.

Herbs for healingsore feet.

Footbath with calendula, chamomile, and peppermint are excellent remedy to heal sore feet.

Warm footbath with calendula, chamomile, and peppermint:

1 cup water

1/2 cup dry calendula flowers, chamomile and peppermint.

2 tablespoons calendula extract

2 teaspoons honey

Boil water, add on dry flowers and steep for 10 minutes. Fill your foot soaking container with warm water, add on the herbal solution and honey, and stir well. Soak your feet for 20-30 min.

Herbs for skin problems.

For itchy skin:

Oatmeal is excellent for your skin, smells good, and leaves your skin feeling soft and fresh. Follow these steps to prepare an easy but effective oatmeal bath to soothe your skin in the comfort of your own home.

- Take plain, unflavored, oatmeal. As optional and additional things you can use lavender buds (about 1/4 to ½ cup) or lavender (or other) essential oils. Milk, butter milk and Epsom salts are other optional and additional things which can be used here.
- Pour about ⅓ to ¾ cup of oatmeal into a bowl, add extras (lavender) if you want. Mix it all up.
- Put the mixture into the coffee filter bag or muslin piece.
- Tie it off with a rubber band, string, or ribbon. Rubber band is the easiest to use.
- Fill the tub with relatively hot water. Add milk (or buttermilk) 1 cup into the tub under the running water. Epsom salts can also be added to ease sore muscles and help achieve softer skin.
- Put the bag with oats into the running water. Allow to cool. As the tub cools to a tolerable temperature, the heat will cause the essences of oatmeal and lavender to disperse.
- Step into the tub when the temperature feels nice for you. Once in the bath, you can gently squeeze the oatmeal sachet to release more of the oatmeal liquid through the bath. Enjoy the bath for as long as wished, although if you are treating

a skin condition, don't stay longer than 10 minutes to avoid aggravating your skin condition.

Herbs to heal athletic foot.

Calendula feet bath can be used. Take 2 heaped tablespoons of herbs to 1 litre of water. Use it in a foot bath for athletic foot. For other form of yeast infection you can add calendula in your bath.

Herbs for haemorrhoids.

Sitz bath with Calendula: Two heaped double handfuls of fresh or 100 g of dried herbs for one sitz bath. Take sitz bath 15-20 min daily.

To relieve water retention and haemorrhoids:
Nettles tea can help with water retention and improving haemorrhoids and other blood vessel problems. Nettle tea can also help ease leg cramps and other muscles spasms.

To prevent or reduce stretch marks.
Rub into the skin Cocoa Butter, apricot scrub, Lavender oil, Aloe Vera. All these herbs are used externally – applied on the top of stretch marks at least 2 times a day.

To tone the uterus and stimulate contractions
(only use in the 3d trimester).

- Red Raspberry Leaf can be drunk in tea form to induce labour after 38th week of pregnancy.
- Blue Cohosh is good for increasing the tone of your uterus to prepare you for birth.
- Black Cohosh is good to regulate contractions and when closer to the actual birth, encourage strong contractions.
- Cramp Bark helps to increase relaxation during the cervix dilation process.

- Partridge Berry helps to tone, reduce stress and relax your uterus.
- Motherwortcan stimulate the uterus through relaxing.
- Evening Primrose Oil can increase uterine contractions.

Herbs to avoid during pregnancy.

Many herbs are not safe during pregnancy. Some plants may irritate the placenta, cause mutation of the developing foetus and stimulate muscular contractions of the uterus amongst others.

1. **Alkaloids.** These plants constrict blood vessels and can cause an increase in blood pressure. Some of them (for example tea and coffee) are Ok in small amounts and if you don't have problems with hypertension. So, it is always better if you consult your physician about the safety of a particular herb.
   Coffee, Tea, Barberry, Ephedra, Golden Seal, Mandrake, Tobacco, Sanguinaria

2. **Bitters.** These herbs can cause miscarriage and/or birth defects.
   Barberry, Cascara Sagrada, Celandine, Feverfew, Gentian, Golden Seal, Mugwort, Rue, Tansy, Wormwood

3. **Diuretics herbs.** These plants can cause dehydration of the body which is very dangerous for you and the baby.
   Buchu, Horsetail, Juniper Berries, Uva-Ursi (small amount is OK)

4. **Emmenagogues** are herbs which stimulate blood flow in the pelvic area and uterus; some stimulate menstruation and can cause miscarriage.
   Black Cohosh (safe in the last six weeks), Blue Cohosh (safe in the last six weeks), Hyssop, Motherwort (OK in small

doses), Mugwort, Myrrh, Nasturtium, Osha, Parsley, Squaw
Vine (small amounts okay), Pennyroyal, Rue, Sage, Shepard's
Purse, Tansy, Wormwood

5. **Laxatives** cause diarrhoea and increase blood flow to the
   pelvic region and increase chance of miscarriage.
   Aloes, Castor Bean, Barberry, Buckthorn, Cascara Sagrada,
   Coffee

6. **Oxytocic** hers stimulate childbirth, by stimulating uterus
   contractions. These herbs are nor recommended during
   pregnancy but can be used for stimulating labour after
   38 weeks of pregnancy.
   Blue Cohosh, Golden Seal, Black Cohosh, Mistletoe, Blue
   Flag, Uva-Ursi, Cotton, Root Bark

CHAPTER 10.

Pain and Aches Management during Pregnancy

Pains and aches are common during all stages of pregnancy. Many pains and aches are just pregnancy discomforts and don't mean anything dangerous. Common pregnancy pains and aches include: back pains, tender breast, sore feet, carpal tunnel syndrome, sciatica, leg cramps, heartburn and other.

The best approach to cope with pains and aches during pregnancy is to listen to them. Treat your pain not as your enemy but as your friend because pain provides critical information about your body needs during pregnancy.

Since the body does not communicate with words, pain is the only mechanisms to signal that something is wrong.

But some pains can be more serious than others, so to avoid any complications, you should always check with your doctor about the nature of any pains you have during pregnancy.

How do you cope up with your pregnancy aches and pains?

The most common methods to manage these aches and pains are over the counter medications like Paracetamol or Panadol or maybe your doctor prescribed you some specific treatments. Whether these are helping or not, it would be good for you to know how to cope with the pregnancy pains and aches using alternative methods.

These methods that I want to share with you are absolutely safe and can't harm your health or baby. There is nothing to take in or swallow. You'll learn to manipulate your pains using your mind and achieving control over your body mentally. This is possible because pain stems from your brain ... and retraining your brain is often one of the best pain-relieving solutions there is.

A meditation to deal with pain and/or illness.

Did you know that meditation provides greater reductions in pain intensity and pain unpleasantness than medications like morphine?

Yes, you can heal pain during meditation. You can scan your body and repair it with love and subtle body energy.

1. *Sit comfortable in a chair or crossed-leg on the floor.*
2. *Breathe and count to 4: inhale 1, 2, 3, 4 and exhale 1, 2, 3, 4.*
3. *Relax into discomfort. Don't try to change it or rid yourself of it. Simply let the pain be. Gently breathe through any discomfort, fear or struggle. Don't resist the pain. Relax all the muscles. Get to know the geography of your pain. Frame it. Familiarise with it.*
4. *Tune into the discomfort. Notice what colour is it? Texture? Emotions? What temperature is it? Does it move or stay in one place? Does it bring any images? Sounds? Smells?*

Memories? Ask the pain: What can I learn from you? How can I ease my pain?

5. *Focus of the discomfort. Feel it completely. When you inhale breathe all your pain in. Visualise it as a cloud of dark smoke. Let it flow throughout your body, right through the centre of compassion and love.*

6. *Now picture the black smoke dissolving purified by love. When exhale, picture this purification as clear white light. Send the light back to the area of pain. Repeat it: breathe in pain, purify it with love and breathe out white love and compassion. Continue until the pain ceases purified by love.*

This meditation can be very effective for relieving all kinds of pregnancy aches and pains: sore back, sore feet, carpal tunnel, sciatica, headaches and any others.

I always support the idea to listen to your pain and tune into your pain but there are other mental techniques to cope with pain. These techniques are based on the notion that you should distract yourself from your pain.

Some people find them helpful. So, here they are:

Altered focus.

This technique can be very effective for local pains: low back pain, carpal tunnel syndrome or feet pains. It involves focusing your attention on any specific **non-painful** part of your body (hand, shoulder, foot, etc.) and altering sensation in that part of the body. For example, imagine your hand warming up or your foot gets cold (or tingly, or numb). This will take the mind away from focusing on the source of your pain.

Mental anesthesia.

Some people say this is very powerful for any chronic pains. You should imagine that an injection of numbing anesthetic (like the Novocain a dentist uses) is given to you into the area of pain. Similarly, you may then wish to imagine a soothing and cooling ice pack being placed onto the area of pain.

Mental pain reliever.

Can be very useful for non-specific pains – pains all over your body, when you feel that every part of your body is aching. Imagine your brain producing massive amounts of endorphins, your body's natural pain relieving hormones, and having them flood into to the painful parts of your body.

Sensations Transfer.

Use your mind to produce altered sensations, such as heat, cold, anesthetic, in a non-painful hand, and then place the hand on the painful area. Imagine transferring this pleasant, altered sensation into the painful area.

Pain movement.

Mentally move your pain from one area of your body to another, anywhere you think the pain will be easier for you to handle. If you can't take another minute of your leg pain, for example, mentally move the pain up from your leg and into your low back. If you want, then move your pain out of your body and into the air.

It usually takes practice for these techniques to become effective but some people feel the pain eases after the first time doing it. It is also beneficial to use it regularly: every day for about 30 minutes each time. As a beginner, less than 30 minutes is normally not enough to relax and change focus. With practice, you will find that your powers over the pain will increase, and it will take less mental energy to achieve more pain relief.

CHAPTER 11

Meditation for Pregnancy

'As your mind quiets, your body takes over.'
(Deepack Chopra)

Pregnancy is a great opportunity to learn about your mind, body and spirit. Meditation is one of the essential parts of this learning. I would advise you to meditate daily, even twice a day: in the morning and at night before going to bed.

Meditation is one of the most effective ways of dealing with stress. Since pregnancy is a stressful time due to the changes it brings, meditation will be a great tool for you to cope with all these changes.

The basic elements of all meditations are focus, breath and subtle body energy. Every time you meditate you need to place your focus on your breath, a particular part of your body or any other things around you or inside you. You must breathe. And the purpose of any meditation is to feel the subtle body energy which can heal and rejuvenate.

The most common and effective meditations are: focused breathing meditation, progressive muscle relaxation, body scan meditation and loving kindness meditation.

1. **Focused breathing meditation.**
   This is one of the most effective ways to ease muscle tension, lower your heart rate, and help you fall asleep.
   - *Sit in a comfortable position with your back straight. You can also lie down if it's more comfortable for you. After the second trimester or if you're uncomfortable lying on your back, rest on your side with a pillow between your legs for support.*
   - *Breathe slowly through your nose, keeping your mouth closed. Be conscious of your stomach rising as you gradually fill your lungs and diaphragm with air.*
   - *Let the flow of your breath settle into its own natural rhythm while keeping focused and aware during the whole process.*
   - *When your attention begins to wander, gently but firmly bring it back to your breathing.*
   - *Count your breath. On exhalation count "one". The next exhalation count "two" and so on until the count of ten, then start over again. Counting can be stopped once you become better at concentrating and focusing your attention.*

2. **Progressive muscle relaxation.** This technique may take a couple of weeks to master, but once you do, you'll be glad you did. It's like a natural sleeping pill, which you'll really appreciate as your pregnancy progresses and a good night's sleep becomes more and more elusive. Here's how to do it: Lie down on your bed or on the floor and tense your muscles completely…then let them totally relax. Focus on one muscle group at a time and alternate between the left and right side of your body. One possible route is to start by tensing and releasing your hand and forearm muscles, followed by your triceps and biceps,

then your face, chest and shoulders, stomach, legs, and finally, your feet.

3. **Body scan meditation.** The purpose of this meditation is not just to relax, but to bring awareness to any sensations you detect, as you scan your body with your attention on each part of the body in turn. You can call it body awareness. The product of this awareness is a balance of the mind, composure, equilibrium. It means not reacting with either craving for what is pleasant, or aversion for what is not pleasant. It means a form of acceptance, unconditional acceptance of one's own experiences.

It is not a way of getting rid of unpleasant sensations. It is not a way of attracting pleasant sensations or pleasant experiences. It is a way of learning to accept whatever is there and get on with life. Relaxation becomes a by-product of that, because when acceptance is increased, you relax.

How to do body scan meditation?

Meditation: Body Scan during Pregnancy.

Sit in a chair or lie down. Choose a place where you will be warm and undisturbed. Allow your eyes to close gently.

Start by focusing all your attention to your nostrils, and look at the incoming and outgoing breath, as it comes in, as it goes out. Do not judge whether this moment is pleasant or unpleasant. We are learning to be neutral and not reactive.

Now move all your attention to the top of your head. There are millions of sensations on the top of your head that your mind hasn't been sharpened enough to feel. You may feel something if you scan with a larger portion each time, maybe 3 or 4 inches diameter at one time. Don't get stuck up with any sensation, whether pleasant or unpleasant.

If any thought comes, gently push them away. If it's still overpowering, breathe slightly harder. Not too hard, slightly harder.

Then move to the forehead and scan the entire forehead area. Scan the eyebrows. Start with one, continue with the other. Move down to the nose. Look at any sensation on the nose. Move further down to the mouth. Survey the lips. Look at the tongue. Are there any sensations on the tongue? Of course your mouth is closed, or the lips gently parted, but you are breathing through the nose. Look at the chin. Move up to the left cheek, and then move aside to the right cheek.

If you have any sensation, don't get attached to it in any way, just move further. Move up to the left ear, and move aside to the right ear. Now survey the throat area. Any sensation is a sensation, it is an experience. Just observe. It arises to pass away, just to pass away. Same with your thoughts. They arise and pass away if you don't nourish them, feed them with more thoughts.

When you finish with the throat, survey the entire neck area. Then move to the left shoulder, the left arm, left elbow and move to the left wrist and left hand. Then go up to the right shoulder, and survey the entire shoulder. Move down to the right arm, the right elbow, the right forearm, and down to the right wrist and the right hand.

Then move up to the upper chest area. Piece by piece. Keep the same order. Then move down, and survey the entire abdominal area.

Then move up to the upper back area and the lower back area. If any thoughts arrive, push them away and go back *to the awareness of any sensation you are looking at, and move further.*

Move down to the buttocks and survey the entire buttocks area. Start with the left, and once this is surveyed, then move to the right buttock. Move down to the left thigh, and survey the entire thigh down to the left knee. Then move down to the left leg and to the left ankle, until you survey the entire left foot.

Now go up to the right thigh, and survey the entire right thigh, part by part. Keep moving, down to the right knee, the right leg, the right ankle and the right foot.

You have now surveyed the entire body from the top of your head to the tip of your toes. Now start from the tip of your toes and go up back to the top of your head. Start from the left foot and move up to the left thigh. And then the right foot, move up to the right thigh. Then survey the buttocks, and the lower back, the upper back, and then the lower abdomen. Then move tothe chest area: from the upper chest go up to the throat.

From the left hand go up to the left shoulder. From the right hand go up to the right shoulder. Then survey the entire neck area, and then the face, part by part, and the entire scalp area.

And again from the top of the head go down to the tip of your toes. Scan your body entirely, as long as you can give it time.

The longer you practice the better your body awareness will be. Body awareness is the key to healing your body with the power of mind. The whole point of this exercise is to develop balance, equanimity and non-reactivity of the mind.

Reactive mind is the one that brings stress, anxiety and behavioural problems. If reactivity of the mind remains untreated more serious problems and illnesses can occur. And this is what we're trying to heal with the body scan meditation.

4. **Loving–kindness meditation**. Loving-kindness is a meditation, which brings about positive attitude to life and systematically develops the quality of 'loving-kindness acceptance'. It acts as a form of self-psychotherapy, a way of healing the troubled mind to free it from its pain and confusion.

How to do it?

Relax all the tension (if any) in your body, and start focusing all your attention on parts of your body that vibrate with peace. Or just focus on the centre of your chest on what we commonly call the heart area. Focus on your heart.

With each incoming breath, feel the sensations in this part of the body. And with each outgoing breath, feel tingling sensations, pleasant flow of sensations taking more and more space in your body with each exhalation. Now start manifesting the following thoughts.

May I be filled with loving-kindness.

May I be safe from inner and outer dangers.

May I be peaceful.

May I be well in body and mind.

May I be at ease and happy.

Now start visualizing people you love, you care for, and think good thoughts for them. This time with each exhalation, let those sensations, pour out of your body, your chest, your hands, your forehead. Let these sensations go towards these people that you love and care for. Picture this person and carefully recite the phrases:

May you be filled with loving-kindness.

May you be safe from inner and outer dangers.

May you be well in body and mind.

May you be at ease and happy.

Now let these sensations pouring out of your body and your thoughts and be directed towards people who are not so close to you. Maybe those who may have had some conflict with you in the past, or with whom there is potential for conflict in the future. Picture this person and carefully recite the phrases:

May he/she develop awareness of himself/herself.

May he/she develop equanimity, peace and tranquillity.

May he/she be happy and filled with loving-kindness.

May he/she be well in body and mind.

And now share your good will and good thoughts with all beings. No exceptions, near or far, all beings.

May all beings be peaceful.

May all beings be happy, all beings.

Meditation will help you to relax and heal yourself. It helps to communicate with your baby on intuitive level. It energises you, clear your mind and free your spirit.

There are many other specific ways to meditate:

5. **Heart-Centring Meditation.**
   This is another kind of meditation which is good for pregnancy as it evoke relaxation, empowerment and feeling loved.

1. Sit comfortably and close your eyes. Take a few long, deep breaths to relieve tension (count 1, 2, 3, 4 when inhale and 1, 2, 3, 4 when exhale). If the negative thoughts intrude (you know that broken record "I am not good enough, it is not going to work, I am wasting my time and bla, bla, bla) keep concentrating on your breath as best as you can. Feel the air entering your nostrils, going down inside your chest. Expand your belly when you inhale (not the chest), than slowly exhale.

2. Tune in to your heart. Lightly rest your palm over your heart in the mid-chest. This energy centre is the entryway to compassion and spirit.

3. In a relaxed state, inwardly request to connect with a higher power, a force greater then yourself that links you to love. It can be God, a star, a mother, a loved one, a child – whatever stirs you.

4. In your heart area, notice what you intuitively feel, not what you think. You may experience a soothing warmth, comfort, clarity, even bliss. It is love or spirit inside you. From that home base, you can better sense it everywhere. Stay aware of your heart as it opens more and more, infusing you with more love and compassion.

5. Continue focusing on that power inside your heart (God, a star, a mother, a loved one, a child) – this is a sacred force that moves you.
   When you become aware of your heart energy (sacred force), you can use it in different ways: you can send this energy to heal different parts of your body; you can connect with it to your baby or any other people you want to connect with.

6. **Connecting with your baby meditation.**
   1. *Sit comfortably and relax.*
   2. *Take a few deep breaths in and out until you feel the sense of relaxation spread out inside your body.*
   3. *Tune in to your heart. Rest your palm over your heart in the mid-chest.*
   4. *In a relaxed state, inwardly request to connect with a higher power, a force greater then yourself that links you to love.*
   5. *Draw an invisible energetic line from your heart to your belly. This is your love line. Now find your baby inside the uterus and connect your love line to your baby's heart. If you are very relaxed, you may start to feel your baby's heart beat and baby's energy.*
   6. *Send your love to the baby, covering it with the light and bliss. Say "I love you" several times and smile.*
   7. *Hold this connection and continue to smile and enjoy it.*

7. **Happiness Meditation: to be happy and joyful.**
   1. *Sit in a comfortable position with your back straight. Place your hands on your laps. Close your eyes and relax. Take some time to soften any tension in your body and allow yourself to relax.*
   2. *Breathe in and breathe out fully. Breathe with your belly (not chest).*
   3. *Remember one of your happiest moments that really touched you. It can be any moment. Maybe a time when you felt close to someone or were doing something you enjoyed... It can be a place where you felt completely happy... Anything that generate the energy of happiness...*

4. *Notice how you felt during this happy moment without thinking about the details. When you are happy.. Feel the smile coming up.. Allow yourself to smile.. Follow that feeling... And stay with that feeling.. Relaxing and smiling and nothing else..*

5. *Feel how natural that is.. Remember that feeling.. Relaxing and smiling.. Being in the feeling of that moment.. Allow it to happen without thinking how... Smiling and relaxing.. And relaxing even more into the nice feeling... and nothing else..*

6. *Keep relaxing and smiling.. Relaxing even more.. And smiling even more..... Keep relaxing and smiling.. And relaxing into the feeling.. And nothing else.. (15 second pause)*

7. *Stop smiling but keep relaxing.. Relaxing even more.. Notice how you feel.. Keep relaxing and relaxing even more.. And nothing else..*

8. *Now let's feel the difference.. Feel how it is when you smile.. (Repeat three times: steps 4 - 8)*

9. *You can open your eyes and give yourself a moment to relax.*

CHAPTER 12

The Power of Music during Pregnancy

Music has healing power. It has the ability to take people out of themselves for a few hours.

– Elton John

Pregnant women who regularly listen to lullabies, classical music and sounds of nature appeared to be emotionally and mentally healthier than women who don't listen to such music.

Why that? How does this music affect the health?

Research showed that music elicits "a splash" of activity in many parts of the brain. The brain activities evoked by certain kinds of music(lullabies, classical music and sounds of nature) reduce stress and release good chemicals (called endorphins or pleasure hormones) which is healing and rejuvenating for the mind and body.

Listening to music also affects the serotonin level in the brain. Serotonin is the chemical which regulates moods: if you're lack of serotonin in the brain you become depressed. But happy and relaxing music has the ability to raise the serotonin level in the brain. Music also distracts the body from suffering and pain. So this music can be a great pain reliever too.

Research showed that sound of music can affect growing tissues. Classical and soothing music encourages the tissue growth and balances it. Your baby is growing inside you (so its tissues are growing). It is also proven that babies in uterus respond to different music differently. Relaxing music makes the baby relax and noisy music makes him/her startle and increases the baby's heart rate (a sort of anxiety state). So be careful what kind of music you're constantly exposed to when you're pregnant.

Foetus ability to hear music.

Baby's ears begin to form around 8 weeks and become structurally complete at about 24 weeks of pregnancy. Many studies have proved that babies can hear and react to sound from as early as 20 weeks (some studies say that even earlier than that) and begin active listening by the 24th week.

The sense of hearing is the most developed of all senses before birth because it gets exercised more than other senses while in uterus. The studies also have found that:

- Babies respond to the loud sounds by accelerating their heartbeats.
- Babies respond to relaxing music by relaxing the muscles, slowing the movements, closing eyes and sleeping.
- Long exposure to loud noises has been linked to birth defects.
- Exposure to 'white noise' has been linked to premature birth and low weight infants. For example, aJapanese study found that pregnant women who lived near Osaka airport had a greater incidence of premature births and delivered smaller babies.

- Babies remember music they hear in the womb more than a year later.

Mothers' observation showed that playing the same calming music they listened to before the baby was born calms the baby after birth.

Mother's voice is the best music.

Because babies remember the music they hear in the womb for a long time, one of the best kinds of music is the mothers' voice.

Yes, your voice is heard and remembered. So, make sure it sounds nice, beautiful and memorable. Just ask yourself a question:

"In what way I would love to be remembered by my dearest one?"

Think of it and brain storm yourself as it is important for you and your child.

Would you like to be remembered like a soft and nice mother?

Would you like to be remembered like a woman with a beautiful and melodic voice?

Would you like to be remembered like a determined, strong and powerful mother?

Your child first memories are in your hands...

Some of you may be saying, "My voice isn't beautiful. It's awful!" But you shouldn't think like that about yourself. You should start thinking differently about yourself and about your voice. You should love it. There is nothing good or bad about your voice – there is something you love or don't. What you love becomes beautiful, what you don't becomes bad. So learn to love your voice and yourself. Your voice is going to determine how your baby will learn to speak, to sing, to communicate with the world around them.

Tips for improving your voice:

1. Always try to sound loving. Don't be different, be yourself, but LOVING.
2. Every day do "Loving-Kindness" meditation which can help you to be and sound loving. Also it will positively affect your voice because mediation heals chakras (our energy centers) and the 5th chakra is our voice chakra. By healing it through meditation you can improve your voice.
3. Listen to calm, relaxing and loving music.
4. Sing nice and loving songs.
5. Avoid situations where you have to argue and fight.
6. Don't watch violent movies or read books about violence. It can change your voice without you realizing it.

Songs to sing when pregnant.

You can sing any songs you like but avoid aggressive and depressive songs. Sing nursery rhymes, lullabies, love songs, any form of chants, spiritual songs, folklore songs, romances or any happy and relaxing songs you know. The songs that have kind and loving energies are the best for pregnancy.

What is the best music to listen to while pregnant?

Generally, you should listen to the music you like but if you are an expectant mother, it is better if you listen to soothing and joyful music, which will make you calmer and happier. As you share hormones with the fetus, your happiness rub off on the well-being of the unborn baby as well.

Try listening to sounds that traditionally have been used to rejoice in spirit, such as Gregorian, Vedic, Hebrew, Native America, Celtic or Hawaiian chants. Popular artists in this genre include Krishna Das, Deva Premal, Bhagavan Das and Snatam Kaur.

Classical music is proved to be very beneficial for mental health of a mother and brain development of a child. Tchaikovsky, Vivaldi, Bach, Mozart, Chopin, Strauss, Schubert, Mendelsohn... and lots more

There are so many classical composers and their music is different. Look through them and find something you like.

New age and meditational music is great for relaxation, enjoyment, reducing stress and healing. Popular themes in New Age music include space and the cosmos, environment and nature, wellness in being, harmony with one's self and the world, dreams or dreaming and journeys of the mind or spirit. Recommended titles of albums and songs are: Shepherd Moons (Enya), Straight' a Way to Orion (Kitaro), Touching the Clouds (Symbiosis), and One Deep Breath (Bradley Joseph).

Many people believe that listening to some classical music while pregnant make your child smarter. This could be true although there is not enough scientific data to proof that. Just listening to classical music on its own without doing anything else probably will not make your child a genius. But early exposure to classics, plus doing a lot of other things beneficial for baby brain development (early learning, special exercises and good teachers) can make a significant impact on cognitive abilities of your child.

Music to avoid during pregnancy.

Not all kinds of music are good to listen to during pregnancy. Studies show that constant exposure to aggressive, discordant music negatively alters the brains structure. Especially it affects the growing brains.

Chaotic music is not good for the audio-stimulation and development of the baby. Research showed that even plants suffer when exposed to this sort of music.

There are 3 types of music that you must avoid when pregnant. It is Rap, Grunge and Hard Rock.

If you are a fan of these styles of music and you really don't want to give up listening then put on headphones and listen to your heart's content. But your baby should not listen to these kinds of music. It can affect negatively his/her nervous system and brain development. For the time you're pregnant stick to something that is sweet and harmonies. Your baby will thank you.

The other interesting fact about your baby's hearing is that your own heartbeat is the first music rhythm lesson your baby will get. That's why it is important for you to stay calm and relaxed as much as possible during pregnancy as the stress increases your heart rate or even can make it irregular (stress arrhythmia).

Rap, Grunge and Hard Rock normally increase the heart rate of the listeners making the listener stressed. That is the other reason why you should not listen these while pregnant.

CHAPTER 13
Bonding with Your Unborn Baby

'A child spends a short time in mommy's belly but an eternity in her heart.'

Bonding (also known as attachment), is how babies, before and after birth, learn what the world is all about. It's also part of their personality development. When there's a healthy attachment between baby and parent the baby comes to believe that the world is a safe place. This is the beginning of the establishment of trust for the baby. For centuries many cultures have believed that some sort of emotional network operated between mother and baby. For this reason mothers were advised to keep their minds and bodies pure during pregnancy.

Nowadays, prenatal psychology (the science subject that study psychology before birth) has proved that much of what was believed about 'mother-baby connection' during pregnancy was true and not just superstitions. When mother is happy, baby is happy; when mother is anxious, baby is too. And that mother can intuitively communicate with her unborn child using language of love.

To be able to bond with a child in uterus parents should accept the notions that:

- preborn babies can hear
- any sound can stimulate a growing foetus
- preborn baby can sense
- preborn baby may think
- your emotional life has long-term effects on your preborn baby
- understand the stress-hormone link between mother and her baby
- remember that emotions, positive or negative, are more intense during pregnancy.

How to bond with your unborn child.

You need to understand that bonding is important for baby's development and you need to find the time to bond with your little one.

1. Massage your bump. A soothing way to bond with your baby is to gently massage oil into your bump. While massaging your belly, try to visualize your baby and intuitively connect to him/her. Send your love, say nice loving words and feel the energy of love around you and your child.

2. Sing to your baby. Singing lullabies, children songs or any kind and loving songs is a great way to connect with your little one.

3. Talk to your baby. Since babies can recognise the voices of their parents when they are born, saying good morning and good night to your baby each day is a good habit to get into. Sharing your feelings and thoughts with your unborn child can also help to 'humanize' your growing belly.

4. Meditate, including your baby in the picture.

5. Pregnancy yoga can help you to bond. When sit in different yoga poses, visualize two of you connect. Send your love and kindness to the baby.

6. Go swimming. Not only is swimming a safe way to exercise but it gives you a chance to relate to your baby, who's floating in fluid too.

7. Keep a scan picture of your baby close by: at your desk, on the table, near your bed, inside your handbag.

8. Respond to your baby's kicks. When your baby kicks, gently poke back. See if he will kick again in that same spot, kick in another spot, or wait until you become still, at which time he kicks again. Then talk about it, giggle, and continue playing. Some babies play hide-n-seek!

9. Visualize your baby. Anything you do always keep in mind your baby and believe that everything you do is for him/her and with him/her. Feel close to your baby and tune into his/her life in the uterus.

10. Sit and have quiet time with your baby. Just sit in your favourite chair, feet up, rubbing your tummy, and talking about whatever is in your heart.

11. Walking can be a great time when you and your baby are alone and connecting. Going for a stroll gives you space to think about your baby. You can even have a discreet chat with your bump as you go.

12. Let your baby know how much you love him/her. Just say it or write it down in diary.

13. Help daddy bond too. Help the dad-to-be to feel your baby move. Let him know that from 23 weeks your baby can hear sounds outside the uterus. Encourage him to talk and read to your bump. This will help your baby become familiar with his daddy's voice.

Chapter 14

Physical Activity during Pregnancy

Regular physical activity should be an essential part of any healthy pregnancy.

Why do you need to exercise while pregnant?

For one thing, if you don't exercise, you'll become less and less fit as your pregnancy progresses — which will make getting back into shape after delivery an even tougher challenge. For another, exercise helps relieve many pregnancy complaints: low energy, constipation, backache, fatigue, insomnia and feet swelling. Plus, regular exercise can give your emotional state a boost, making you happy and stopping those notorious pregnancy mood swings. It regulates your weight and balances metabolism.

Your baby benefits if you exercise too! Considering that the child's first learning starts in uterus, your exercises will be a great lesson for your baby. It will condition him/her to love physical activity since the time of conception.

The best pregnancy exercises are walking, swimming, dancing, jogging, low impact aerobic and supervised classes such as yoga, Tai chi or Pilates.

Exercise does wonders for you during pregnancy. It helps prepare your body for childbirth by strengthening your muscles and building endurance.

Your body releases a hormone called relaxin during pregnancy which loosens your joints in preparation for delivery, so you need to take care with the choice of exercise and pay attention to technique. It's important to find exercises that won't injure you or harm the baby.

It is the best if pregnancy exercises include such important elements as: breathing, stretching and strengthening core muscles (pelvic floor muscles).

Core exercises train the muscles in your pelvis; lower back, hips and abdomen to work in harmony. This helps you to cope with many pregnancy complaints, make the labour easier and the postpartum smoother.

If you haven't started doing core muscles exercises yet, don't worry! Here you can look at the set of pregnancy "Core muscles strength" exercises, deliberately designed for pregnant women. These exercises also involve breathing elements as deep breathing is especially important for pregnant women. Not only it is relaxing (reduces stress), it can also improve your body awareness and teach you to control your breath — which is especially helpful for coping with labour pain. Most people typically take shallow breaths from the upper chest. Breathing deeper allows your lower abdomen and lungs expand fully, providing better gas exchange and more oxygen to the baby.

"Core muscles strength" exercises.

1. Stand upstraight; put your hands together in front of your chest. Centre yourself by taking a few deep breaths in and out. Slowly lift yourself up on to your tiptoes and raise your hands up (take a slow breath in). Stretch yourself. Then

slowly lower your body and sit on your heels, bending your head to the floor (and exhale). Lift yourself up and stand in starting position (breath in). Repeat 7 times.

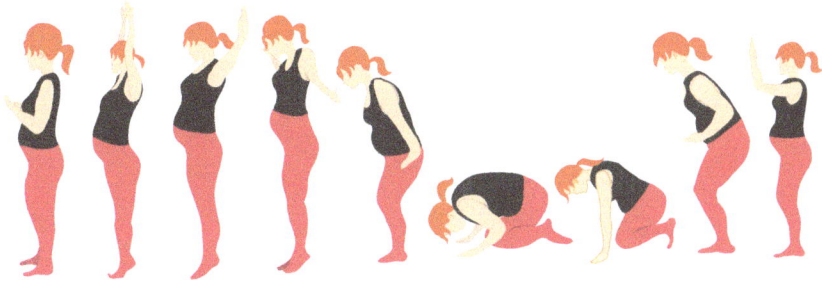

2. "The wave" exercise. Sit on your heels (inhale). Keep your hands down. Bend your body forward then round your back. Move your arms forward and stretch them (exhale). Then return to the starting position: sit on your heels with your hands on your thighs (inhale). Repeat 'wave' like movement 7 times.

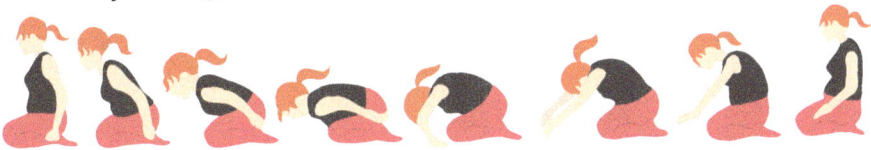

3. "Cat stretching back" exercise. This exercise improves flexibility of the spine, low abdomen and buttocks. Get down on your hands and knees, round your back and do "wave-like" movements of your body - back and forth, imagining yourself a cat. Inhale when the body is lengthening and exhale when the body is shrinking. Repeat 7 times.

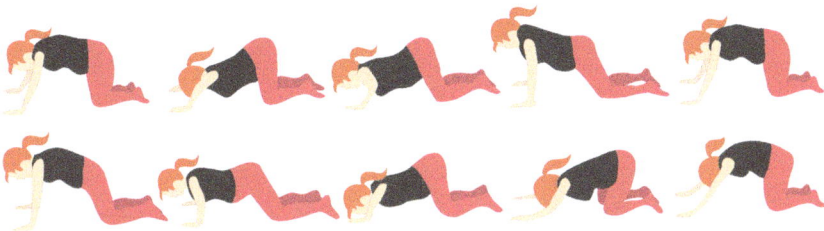

4. Get down on your hands and knees. Lift one leg up and back (inhale). Put the leg down (exhale). Do the same with the other leg. Repeat 5-7 times with each leg.

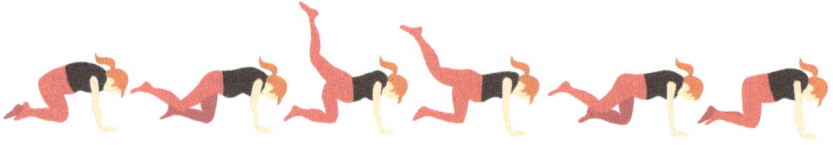

5. Stand up straight; put your feet shoulder width apart. Rotate shoulders back. When the right shoulder goes up – inhale. When the right shoulder is down – exhale.

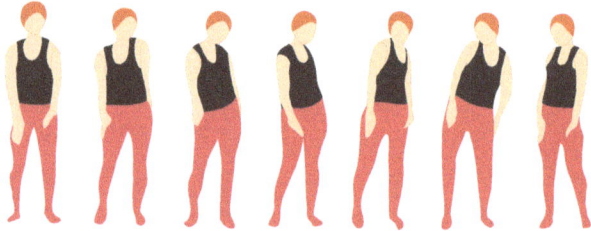

6. Stand up straight; put your feet together. Move your arms out and forward at a shoulder level, then swing them up and back as far as possible stretching your chest (inhale). Then spread your arms sidewise and put them down (exhale). Go back to the starting position. Repeat 7 times.

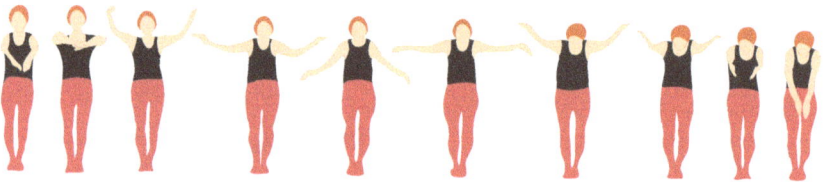

7. "The wave" exercise from a standing position. Stand up straight and put one foot a step forward. Stretch your arms out and slowly bend your body forward (inhale). Create "the wave" like movement of your body and arms: forward and back (exhale). The same is repeated with the other leg a step forward. Repeat 7 times.

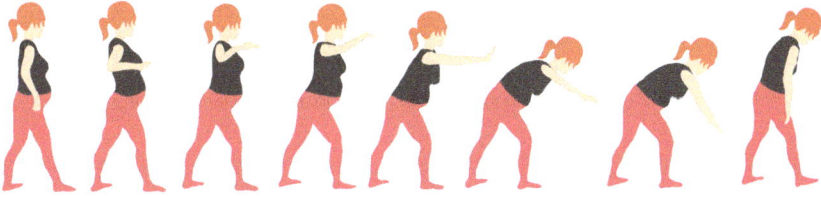

8. Standup straight; put your feet shoulder width apart. Slowly rotate your body clockwise 5 times. Then, do the same but anticlockwise 5 times. Inhale when the body is bent forward and exhale when the body is bent back.

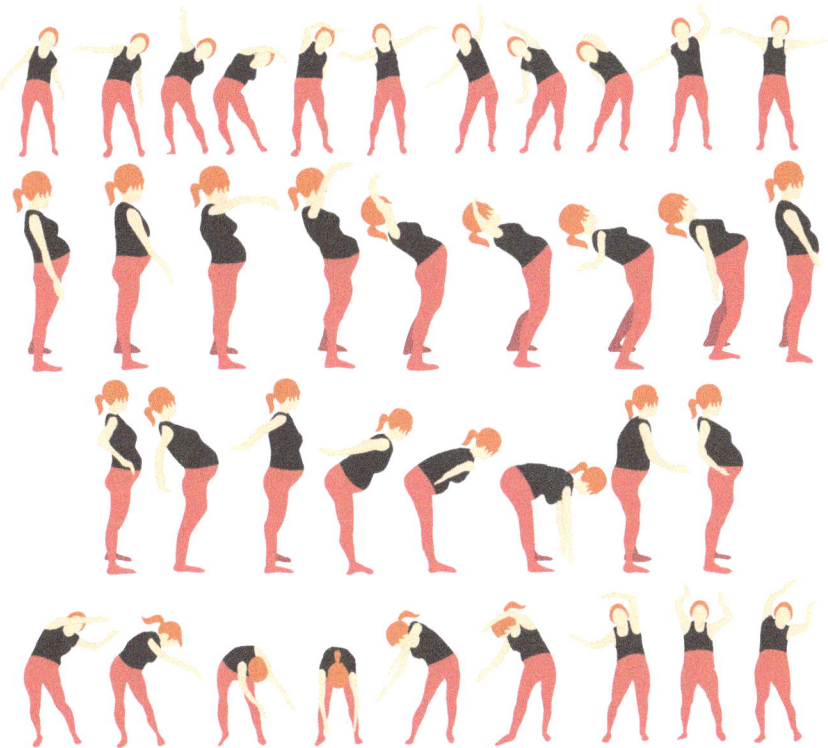

9. Stand up straight; put your locked hands on the forehead. Tilt your head forward, while creating resistance with your hands. Then, put your locked hands on the back of your

head and bend your head back while creating resistance with your hands. Then tilt your head right and left creating resistance with your hands.

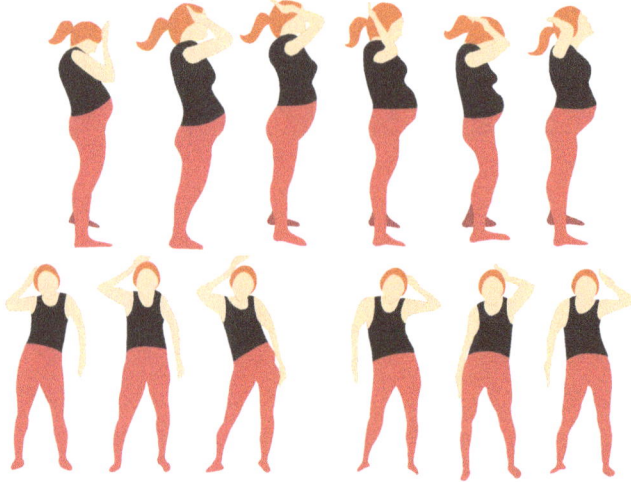

10. Stand up straight. Tilt your head right and left. Then turn your head to the left and to the right. Then make circular movements of the head. Repeat 7 times.

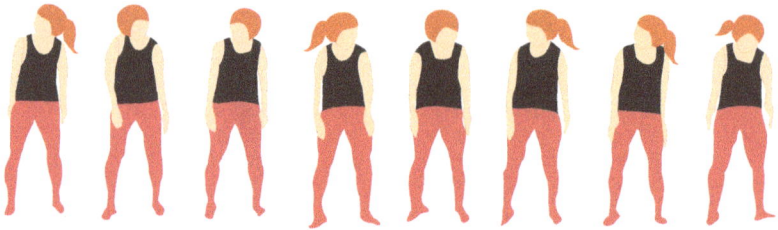

11. Get down on your hands and knees; your eyes look at the floor. Perform push-ups. If possible make push-ups not from knees but from the feet. Inhale when go down, exhale when go up. Repeat 10 times.

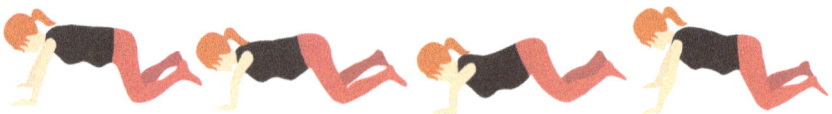

12. Get down on your hands and knees. Lift one leg and make circular movements at the hip joint. Then swing the leg back and sideways. Do the same with the other leg. Repeat 10 circles with each leg.

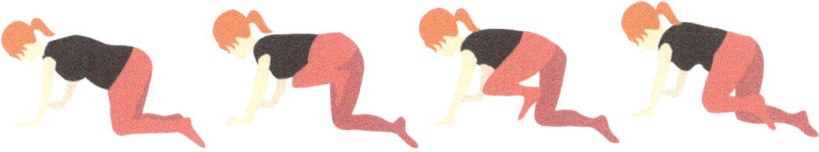

13. Stand up straight; put your feet shoulder width apart. First, lift one leg and rotate it at the hip joint. Then do kicking forward, backward and sideways. Change leg and do the same movements with the other leg.

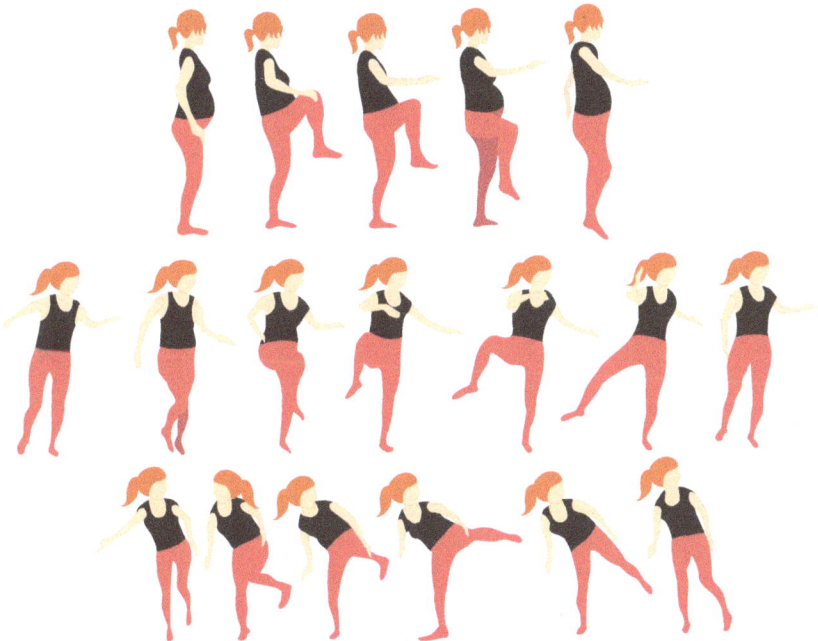

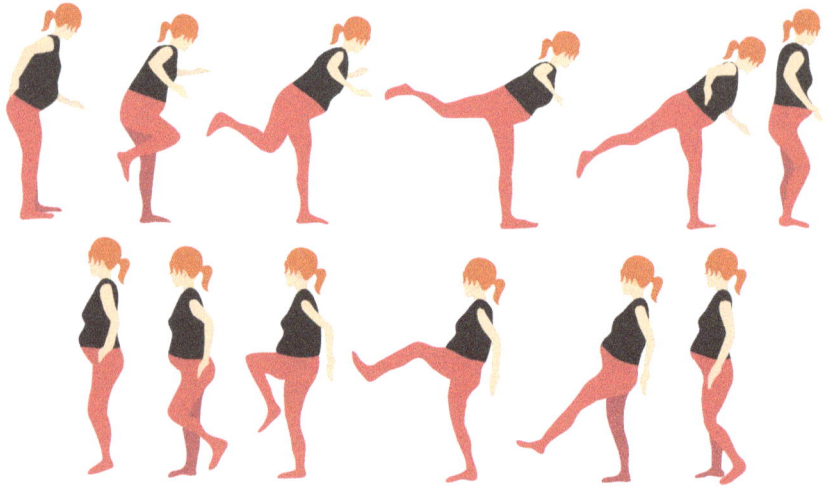

14. Lie on your back. Your hands are behind your head. Lift your legs and torso at the same time. Stretch your arms forward and balance on your bottom until counting 10. Slowly lie down. Repeat 5 times.

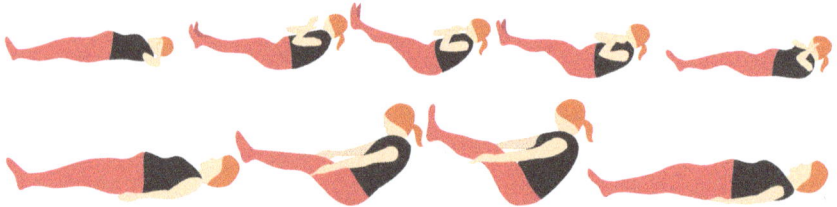

15. Lie down on your back and throw your legs over your head trying to touch the floor with your toes. (This exercise is for the 1st and 2nd trimester only).

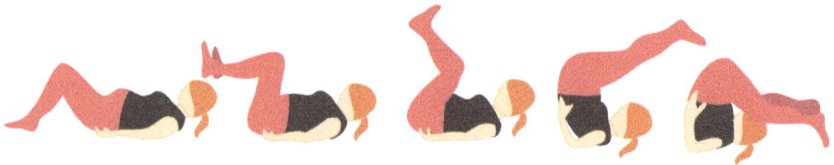

16. "Tree" position. Lie down on your back. Slowly raise your legs and tor soup, supporting your back with your hands, hold this position for count 5, and then slowly put your legs down.(This exercise is for the 1st and 2nd trimester only).

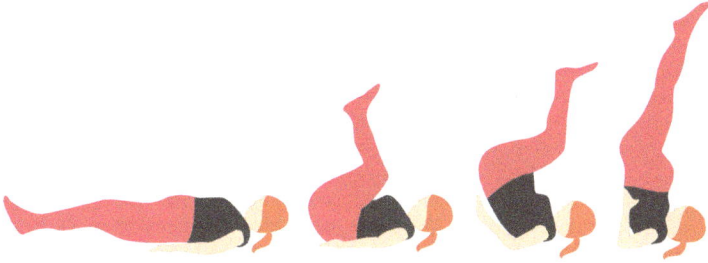

17. Lie on your back, knees bent and feet apart. Raise and lower your pelvis and back. When your pelvis is up, squeeze your pelvic floor muscles and relax them when put the pelvis down. Inhale when rising and exhale when lowering the back. Repeat 10 times.

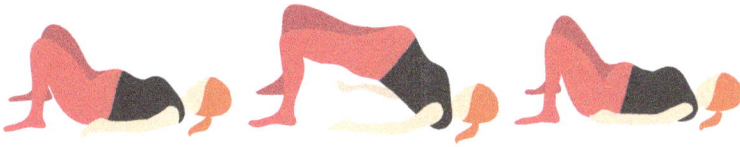

18. Butterfly pose: sit on the floor keeping feet together and knees spread apart as much as possible. Try to lower your knees to the floor. You can help with your hands. Keep the pose for 2-3 min.

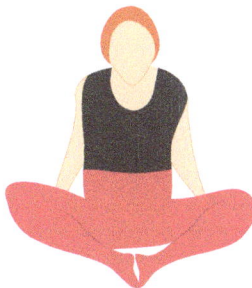

19. "Tiger walk". Try to imitate the walk of a tiger. Your hands should depict the movements of the front paws.

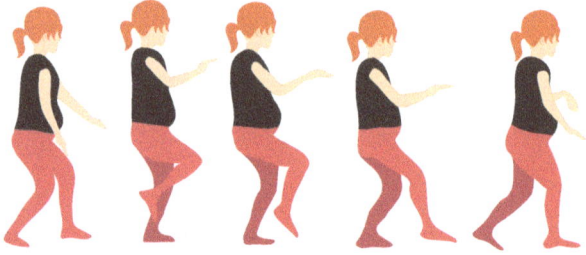

21. "Bear walk". Try to imitate the walk of a bear. Elevate your legs and sway them around when making steps. Waddle around like a bear.

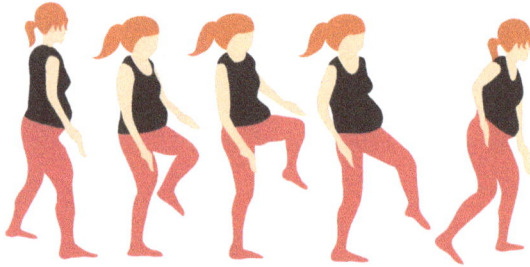

22. Go jogging for 1-2 min.

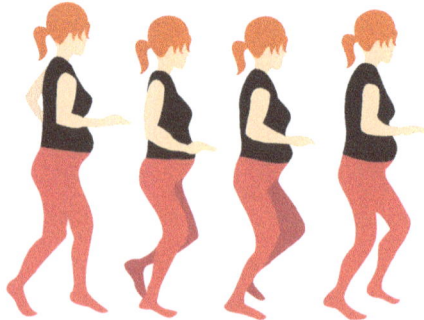

23. "Flying Bird". Wave your arms as if these are wings. Walk around in circles. Inhale when the arms go up; exhale when the arms go down.

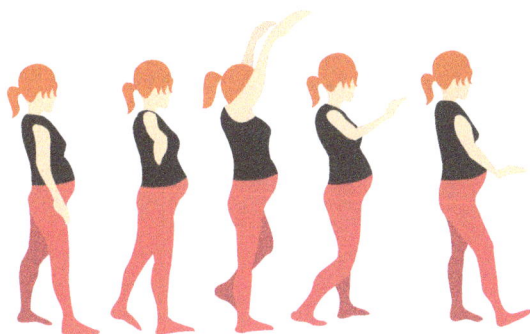

24. Stand up straight; put your feet a bit wider than shoulder width apart. Squat, spreading the knees wide apart and touching the floor with your hands. Stand up. Inhale when standing up and exhale when squatting. Repeat 10 times.

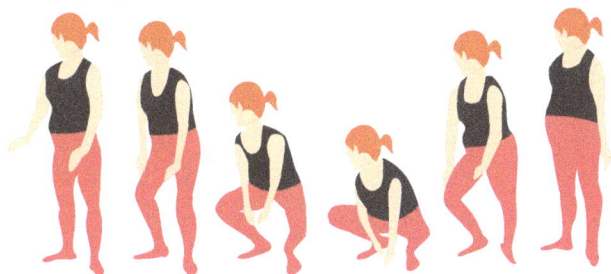

25. Sit on one leg, the other leg straightened to the side. Then transfer the body weight to the other leg. You can do the body transferring with or without help of your hands. Repeat 7 times.

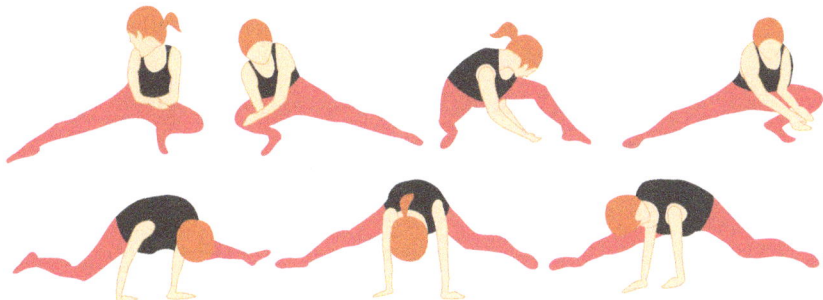

26. Stand up straight; feet slightly apart, eyes closed. Focus on your breathing for 3-5 min. Give gratitude for your health, your body and your ability to exercise. Thanks God (Universe or Divine) for your pregnancy and for your ability to give a new life.

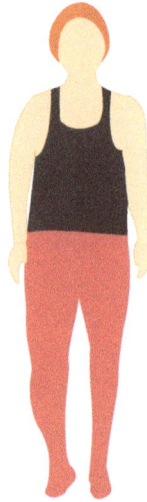

Special Pregnancy Exercises that Help Prevent and Treat Pregnancy Problems.

There are some special exercises you can do at home to prevent or even treat certain pregnancy problems.

1. **Kegel exercises** are also called pelvic floor exercises because they can treat and prevent pelvic floor weakness. The pelvic floor is a "hammock" of muscles that hold the pelvic organs in place. Kegel exercises are important to do before, during and after pregnancy.

Benefits of Kegel exercises.

They strengthen the pelvic floor muscles, which support the uterus, bladder, small intestine and rectum. That means that by doing Kegels you can prevent and treat urinary incontinence, fae-cal incontinence, haemorrhoids, vaginal prolapse, uterus prolapse and many other problems related to weakening of pelvic floor mus-cles. Many factors can weaken your pelvic floor muscles, including pregnancy, childbirth, surgery, aging and being overweight.

Also, Kegel exercises:

- Make labour easier by training the right muscles.
- Improve sexual function by increasing the sensations during intercourse.
- Help to control the muscles inside your body.

Pelvic floor muscles do not get exercised during normal every-day activities and conventional exercise programs. They need special attention. But a good news is that Kegel exercises are easy to do and can be done anywhere without anyone knowing.

How to do Kegel exercises

First, you need to identify the right muscles. While urinating, try to stop the flow. This tightening is the basic move of Kegels. For exercising, don'tdo it while urinating (it is to identify the right muscles only) as doing Kegels while urinating can actually have the opposite effect, weakening the muscle. Do Kegels any time of the day but not when urinating.

The other way to identify the right muscles is to place your finger in your vagina and squeeze your muscles. You should feel the muscles tightening and your pelvic floor move up. Relax and you'll feel the pelvic floor move back again.

Muscles tightening and relaxing is what you need to do for Kegels. Do these movements up to 100-200 times a day. You can do them any time: while waiting in a queue, in a doctor's office, while watching TV or reading a book.

The optimal technique of Kegel is: squeeze for 3 seconds and then relax for 3 seconds.

Repeat this exercise in different session during a day. Kegel exercises are only effective when done regularly. The more you exercise, the more it will be effective.

Exercises for Varicose Veins relieve.

Varicose veins affect about one in three women. You're more likely to get them if they run in the family or if you are overweight. Pregnancy aggravates the condition.

Fortunately, you can prevent or improve the existing condition by doing special exercises. Of course, you must do it on a regular basis and be consistent while doing it.

The exercises we are offering here, improve blood circulation – especially the upward flow. You can do all of them or choose those you like the most. Remember that regularity is the key to success.

Walking:

The simplest exercise is to walk more. Get your legs moving. Walking is a great way to encourage blood circulation in your legs. Instead of taking the elevator or escalator use the stairs. Even going for a short walk around the block before going to work is enough to vastly improve symptoms.

Pedalling:

Lie on the floor, flat on your back. Place your hands out to your sides. Lift your legs off the floor, and pedal them as if you were pedalling a bicycle. The more you elevate your legs, the more you will increase blood circulation. Reversely keeping your legs lower will increase resistance on your abdominals, toning your stomach. Continue this exercise until you feel the blood circulating through your legs and any existing pain has begun to abate.

Pelvic Tilt:

Vigorous 'pelvic tilting' during pregnancy can improve the blood flow from your legs to your upper body.

Stand with your feet shoulder-width apart and your hands on your hips. Slowly tip your pelvis forward, then backward, gradually increasing speed until you are swinging your hips forward and back vigorously. You can also roll and rock your hips and make figure-eights in belly-dancer fashion. Do this for 5-10 minutes a day.

Leg Lifts:

Lie on your back, placing your hands beneath your buttocks to eliminate lower back strain. Lift one leg at a time and hold in an elevated pose perpendicular to the floor. Hold this pose until you feel the blood begin to flow back up from your feet, your calves, and your thighs. Repeat the motion with your other leg. For ultimate relaxation, lie on the floor with your buttocks almost touching a wall. Rest both your legs in an elevated pose resting against the wall, and feel the circulation in your legs improve. Alternately, you can raise both legs and rotate your ankles to further improve leg circulation.

Knee bends with ankle flexion:

Lie again on the floor on your back. Slowly pull one knee into your chest, holding onto your leg behind your knee. While your leg is in this position, point and flex your foot several times. Do this slowly and forcefully, feel the muscles of the calves and the tendons around your ankle tightened. Repeat with the opposite leg.

Exercises for Back Pain.

Rounding and flattening your back.

Get down on your hands and knees and round your back while holding in your abdominal muscles. Continue to breathe while holding this position for count of 10. Release your muscles by flattening your back, but be careful not to make your back concave. Repeat 12 times. Since backaches can last long after childbirth, you can continue to do this exercise even after delivery if you find it helpful.

Pelvis tilts (all variations) are also helpful for reliving back pain.

What exercises to avoid during pregnancy?

Avoid physical activities that involve high risk of falling and damaging the belly. These include horseback riding, downhill skiing, waterskiing, cycling (1st trimester is OK but not 2nd and 3d trimester), all contact sports, diving and scuba diving, sprinting, aerobic exercise in high altitudes, and calisthenics that are not designed for pregnancy. (read chapter "What to avoid during pregnancy")

Chapter 15

Body Care during Pregnancy

Pregnancy hormones can affect almost every part of your body, including your breasts, skin, hair, teeth, and gums. To keep your body in good shape, you'll probably need to make some changes in your daily routine.

Skin care.

During pregnancy it is normal to experience some skin changes. Most of them are due to pregnancy hormones and altered metabolism. Pregnancy related skin changes are not dangerous and most of them go away after birth. With good skin care you can significantly minimize the unwanted changes and protect your skin. So, what are they – common pregnancy skin conditions?

Chloasma is brown patches of pigmentation on the forehead, cheeks, and neck. On darker skinned women, they appear as lighter patches. It's caused by the increased production of melanin, the tanning hormone, which protects the skin against ultra-violet light.

What can you do to help?

Stay out of the sun as much as possible and wear a sunscreen of at least SPF 15 (sunlight can also intensify hyper pigmentation). A hat and long sleeves are a good idea if you're fair-skinned, heading to the beach, or have a historically sensitive complexion. You can use a good concealer to cover particularly pesky spots, but skip bleaches or other chemically based lightening treatments until after you give birth. No peels or lasers, either.

Natural facial masks with yogurt, honey and lemon may help with pigmentation problem during pregnancy.

Yogurt, Honey and Lemon Facial Mask.

Prepare the mixture: 1 table spoon of natural yogurt and 1 tea spoon of runny honey and a few drop of lemon. Apply to face. Let sit for 15-20 minutes. Wash face with steaming washcloth.

For dry skin, use an extra honey. For oily skin a few drops of fresh lime juice.

Linea nigra (dark line running up your tummy). It normally appears around the second trimester and is caused by pigmentation in the skin where your abdominal muscles stretch and slightly separate to accommodate your growing baby.

Both chloasma and lineanigra and other skin discolorations appear to get worse if you don't take enough folic acid. So make sure to take folate as a supplement and eating foods rich in folates when you pregnant.

Glowing skin. The increased volume of blood causes the cheeks to take on an attractive blush, because of the many blood vessels just below the skin's surface. On top of this redness, the increased secretions of the oil glands give the skin a waxy sheen.

Spider veins. These tiny clusters of broken capillaries (small blood vessels), or spider naevi as they are sometimes known, most often appear on the cheeks, and can be found anywhere on the skin during pregnancy.

Spots and acne. The production of sebum, the skin oil, is higher during pregnancy due to high hormones levels. Too much sebum causes pores to become blocked, resulting in greasy skin and spots.

Natural Masks for Better Skin during Pregnancy.

Natural masks are the best remedies to combat facial skin problems during pregnancy. General rules to follow when applying a face mask are:

- Pull back hair, pin it up, tie it, just make sure they are out of the way.
- Clean your face before applying the mask.
- Always apply with fingertips. Apply it over the forehead, cheek, nose, chin and neck.
- Never apply the mask around the eye area. The eye area is really sensitive, so leave it free of mask.
- Try to relax when you have put the mask on, try not to talk, and lie down. The best time to apply a mask is when you are soaking in a bathtub.
- Leave on the mask for the recommended period of time, and not longer.

Egg and Almond oil Facial Mask for Dry skin.

Beat 1 egg and add 1 teaspoon of almond oil to it and mix it thoroughly and apply it on the face evenly and leave it on for around 10-15 minutes. Rinse it off after that with cold water.

Cucumber Yogurt Facial Mask for Oily and Combination Skin.

Make a puree of ½ a cucumber and 1 tablespoon yogurt in a blender and apply it on the face evenly. Leave it on the face for 10-15 minutes and then wash it off with cold water.

Cornmeal Facial Mask for all Types of Skin.

Take enough cornmeal which will be required for the face and mix it with water. Make a thick tight paste and apply it in circular motions to the face and then leave it on for 10-15 minutes or till it dries completely on the face and once it dries wash it off with cold water.

Banana Honey Yogurt Facial Mask for all Types of Skin.

Mash a banana thoroughly and mix it with 1 teaspoon honey and 2 teaspoons yogurt and apply it on the face evenly. Leave it on the face till the skin absorbs it thoroughly and dries completely on the face and then rinse it off with cold water.

Avocado Facial Mask for Dry and sensitive skin.

Mash half an avocado and apply it on the face thoroughly everywhere and let it stay till it dries up completely and then wash it off with cold water.

Apple Facial Mask for All types of skin.

Take a nicely ripe 1/4th apple and mash it with a fork and add 1 teaspoon oatmeal and 1 teaspoon honey to it and apply it on the face and leave it on till the mixture dries on the face thoroughly and then rinse it off with ordinary water.

Honey Mask for all Types of Skin.

The best facial mask is honey, because it helps to open the pores and clean the face. It should be first rinsed off with luke-warm water and then with cold water to close the pores since the pores should be closed after cleansing. Application of facial masks is a must to open the pores in the skin and to remove the dirt and grit inside the skin and close it thereafter.

Stretchmarks. They affect over 90 per cent of pregnant women and may appear as you put on more weight during pregnancy, causing the skin to stretch.

Chafing. As you put on weight, chafing can take place between your thighs or under your breasts, resulting in red, moist skin. Your skin may then become inflamed and blistered and you may notice an odour.

What can you do to help?

Chafed skin will heal faster if it is left uncovered and allowed to breathe. While this may not be possible during the day, make sure that your sleepwear is loose and comfortable so that your skin can get some "airtime" while you snooze.

Wear loose fitting shorts, preferably knit, such as long gym shorts. What causes chafing is your upper thigh rubbing against the material in the clothing you're wearing. It's not something you really notice until it's too late.

Thoroughly rinse the soap from your clothes. And it is recommended not to use strong detergents or heavily perfumed fabric softeners. These products can cause skin irritation and make the chafing even worse.

Use Vaseline to soothe the affected area. It helps to keep the skin slippery, which allows the skin on the legs for example, to slip past each other, rather than rub against each other. These treatments can be really inexpensive, yet they are also really effective.

Sensitive, irritated skin. Skin tends to become more sensitive during pregnancy, not only due to higher hormone levels, but because it has become more stretched and delicate.

What can you do?

Use moisturizers that are water-based. Avoid greasy products and lanoline – they will block your pores.

It is always better to care of your skin with home remedies if you haven't found products that are good for your skin. Olive oil and Aloe Vera gel acts as cleanser. Almond oil and jojoba oil acts as a moisturizer.

Once in a week apply oatmeal mask - take 1 tablespoon of oatmeal powder, egg white or yogurt and mix well. Spread the mixture on the face. Let it dry for at least 20 minutes and wash your face with warm water.

Take egg white mix well and apply over your face. Let it dry and wash your face with warm water.

Scrubbing is one of the best ways to exfoliate dead skin. It is always better and safe to use homemade scrub for sensitive skin as beauty products may be too harsh.

Homemade scrub with baking soda.

Take 2 tablespoons of baking soda add ½ teaspoon of salt and 1 tablespoons of water, mix everything thoroughly. Use the paste as a scrub and wash your face with warm water. Follow this method once in 15 days. Avoid frequent usage as it may damage the skin.

Rinsing face with vinegar solution.

Vinegar is the best homemade medicine for sensitive skin. Add 4 drops of vinegar in half a bucket of bathing water; this will help your skin from soap alkalis. Always avoid steam during facials.

For itchy spots.

For itchy spots, a dab of calamine lotion should help. If any rash or irritation lasts longer than a couple of days, ask your practitioner about next steps. Avoid products that are laden with tons of additives, dyes, or fragrance, any of which can exacerbate the problem.

Protect your skin from the sun.

Always protect your skin from the sun with a high-factor sunscreen (SPF 15 or more). Keep your body well moisturized.

What to avoid for sensitive skin?

Long soaks in the tub can dry out your skin, so keep baths short or switch to showers. Lay off the soap — use a gentle nonsoapy cleanser, keep face washing to a minimum, and use unbleached all-cotton towels and washcloths. Skip fragranced lotions and potions for now as well.

Rashes and itchiness. Hormonal changes make you more sensitive to contact with substances that would not normally affect you. You can become sensitive to chlorine in the swimming pool. One of the common causes of itchiness during pregnancy is thrush.

Thrush remedies:

1. Use live probiotic in adequate amounts to prevent thrush from growing.
2. Taking garlic internally is one of the most effective, quick ways to rid thrush for many women.
3. Do not douche or you may further upset the flora balance in your vagina, as you'll not only wash away the bad bacteria but the good bacteria too.
4. Avoid underwear that is tight or contains materials like lycra and other fabric which reduces air circulation – cotton is best. Avoid underwear wherever possible – not a good idea though if you are going to work and wear a short skirt! Around the home and overnight is a good start.
5. Avoid tight jeans or trousers where possible – opt for skirts if you can.
6. Candida albicans thrive in moist, warm environments so try to avoid long, hot baths and dry yourself properly afterwards.
7. Good old Gentian Violet (water base) is still extremely effective for vaginal thrush.
8. Try avoiding yeast – lot of women swear that yeast in their diet increases the growth of candida.
9. High levels of sugar in diets seems to be a very common culprit, look to amending the diet – cut out soft drinks,

processed foods, breads and pastries – anything that we well know is not good for us.

Intense itching. Intense itching all over, but particularly on your hands and feet, can be a sign of a rare liver disorder that only occurs in pregnancy - obstetric cholestasis. This condition should be treated by a doctor. Call to your doctor as soon as you can.

General help: keeping cool might help to ease the itch. You can try things like: lowering the temperature in your house, keep your body uncovered at night, take cool showers and baths, soak your feet or hands in ice water. A bland moisturiser cream may also give some temporary relief from itch.

Hair Care during Pregnancy.

Pregnancy brings many changes to your hair. Your hair can become thicker as higher oestrogen levels slow your hair's shedding process, so hairs that would normally fall out stay on your scalp, thickening your locks. Straight hair might get a bit of bounce or even full-fledged curls; curly hair might go straight. You might find changes in the moisture levels of your hair along with changes in its texture. If you're lucky, your hair might move in the direction you want. But anything can happen.

Enjoy the change while it lasts, and simply modify your hair-care routine during pregnancy — your hair is likely to return to its normal state after your baby is born.

Consider waiting until the second trimester for hair dye, bleaching, permanents or straightening. Don't dye or bleach eyebrows or eyelashes while pregnant. This could cause swelling or increase risk of infection in the eye area.

Natural aids for hair care during pregnancy.

During pregnancy try to use only natural treatments for your hair. Eggs, yogurt and honey are great components for hair treatments during pregnancy. And they're not the only ones. There are many natural products that are better for your hair then any expensive beauty products. These are avocado oils, lemon juice, baking soda, raw eggs and much more.

Egg treatment for all hair types.

For normal hair, use the entire egg to condition hair; use egg whites only to treat oily hair; use egg yolks only to moisturize dry, brittle hair.

Use ½ cup of whichever egg mixture is appropriate for you and apply to clean, damp hair. If there isn't enough egg to coat scalp and hair, use more as needed. Leave on for 20 minutes, rinse with cool water (to prevent egg from "cooking") and shampoo hair. Whole egg and yolks-only treatments can be applied once a month; whites-only treatment can be applied every two weeks.

Dairy products treatment for dull hair.

Massage ½ cup sour cream or plain yogurt into damp hair and let sit for 20 minutes. Rinse with warm water, followed by cool water, then shampoo hair as you normally would. Treatment can be applied every other week.

Lemon juice and olive oil mixture for itchy scalp.

Mix 2 tablespoons fresh lemon juice, 2 tablespoons olive oil and 2 tablespoons water, and massage into damp scalp. Let mixture sit for 20 minutes, then rinse and shampoo hair. Treatment can be applied every other week.

Beer treatment for limp or fine hair.

Mix ½ cup flat beer (pour beer into a container and let it sit out for a couple of hours to deplete carbonation) with 1 teaspoon light oil (sunflower or canola) and a raw egg. Apply to clean, damp hair, let sit for 15 minutes, then rinse with cool water. Treatments can be applied every other week.

Honey treatment for dry or sun-damaged hair.

Massage approximately ½ cup honey into clean, damp hair, let sit for 20 minutes, and then rinse with warm water. You can also add 1 to 2 tablespoons olive oil to loosen the honey for easier application. For extremely sun-damaged hair, mix honey with 1 to 2 tablespoons of a protein-rich ingredient, like avocado or egg yolk. Treatment can be applied once a month.

Cornmeal or corn starch for oily or greasy hair.

Pour 1 tablespoon cornmeal or corn starch into an empty salt or pepper shaker and sprinkle onto dry hair and scalp until you've used it all. After 10 minutes, use a paddle hairbrush to completely brush it out. Treatment can be applied every other day.

Avocado for frizzy hair.

Mash up half an avocado and massage into clean, damp hair. Leave it for 15 minutes before rinsing with water. You can add on 1 - 2 tablespoons of a hydrating ingredient, like sour cream, egg yolks or mayonnaise to the mixture. Treatment can be applied every two weeks.

Baking soda for residue-ridden hair.

Mix 1 to 2 tablespoons baking soda with small amounts of water until a thick paste forms. Massage into damp hair and let sit for 15 minutes. Rinse with water, and then shampoo hair. Treatment can be applied every two weeks.

Tooth and Gum Care.

Gum problems are common in pregnancy. Your gums may bleed when you brush or floss them. The hormone progesterone softens your gums and increases the blood supply to them. The plaque, which coats your teeth between cleaning, also make your gums more prone to bleeding.

What can you do?

- Brush your teeth twice a day for at least two minutes (not for 20 seconds, as most people). When brush your teeth do it with small circular motions, gently brushing the gums as well. Don't brush too vigorously. It often causes gum problems. Electric toothbrushes can tackle this by preventing hard pressing.
- Floss every night. Brushing does not remove the plaque between teeth and by the gum line. If you don't floss, you leave about 35% of the surface of your teeth uncleaned.
- Use mouthwash to complete the cleaning. The following simple natural mouthwash will help you to promote teeth and gums health:

    1 glass of water

    1 tea spoon of baking soda or sea salt

    2-3 drops of essential oil (tea tree oil, chamomile oil, peppermint oil, thyme oil, lemon oil, or sage oil).
- Eat at least an apple every day. Apples are great for teeth cleaning and strengthening.

CHAPTER 16

Love Your Changing Body

Some women welcome their pregnant bodies, while others are in complete shock over the different changes. Natural changes are inevitable during pregnancy as hormone fluctuations will cause your uterus to expand, your breasts to grow, your feet to enlarge, and your skin to break out. You may suffer increased fatigue and incredible food cravings.

Loving your body before pregnancy usually helps you get through the physical and emotional changes of pregnancy. Changing your body image while you are pregnant is harder.

Here are some ideas to try and help you love and accept your pregnant body:

- Understand and accept the spiritual aspect of pregnancy. See your body as a place where you and your baby live.
- Realize that without your body, both of you can't survive. So you must love your body and nurture it as a hospitable home for two of you.
- Focus on your baby. Your body is changing in order to help your baby grow and develop. It is a natural process.
- Express your feelings. Talk with your partner, family, or friends about how you are feeling. Keeping your feelings bottled up will only make you feel worse.

- Get more enjoyment from exercise, walking and swimming. Enjoyment brings more satisfaction and pleasure. As a consequence, loving feelings will grow.
- Do yoga and meditation daily. These practices focus on the link between your body and mind. Love grows when mind and body are connected.
- Practice self-massage. Touching your own body will help you to become more familiar and accepting of it.
- Learn as much as you can about pregnancy. By educating yourself, you will know what to expect and feel more in control.

Mistakes to avoid:

1. **Don't compare your pregnancy to another woman's.** Every pregnancy is different; every baby is different. You may gain more or less weight during pregnancy than other women. Different factors contribute to this such as: the size of your baby, your physical fitness, how much you exercise, if you have bed rest or not, your age, the difficulty of your pregnancy and birth, having a multiple birth, the time of year you're pregnant, your support system, how many other children you have, whether or not you work outside the home. And the list can go on and on. The main point here is to have compassion for the unique circumstances that affect you and your body. Release the expectation that your experience – and your body – should be like everyone else's.

2. **Don't compare your current pregnancy with previous pregnancies.** The same reason is applied here: different circumstances bring different pregnancy. You can gain little amount of weight during your first pregnancy but become quite heavy during your second pregnancy. Or vice versa.

Don't criticize yourself for that as different circumstances surrounded this pregnancy and you can't be responsible for them. Treat yourself with compassion and gratitude. Always thank your body for providing a good place for you and your baby to live in.

3. **Don't compare yourself to celebrities.** This can be quite dangerous because if you start comparing yourself with the modern celebrities, you put yourself up against something unachievable for a normal person. Achieving this goal involves lots and lots and lots of work, money, good genes, and loads of support from professionals (everything from a nanny to a personal trainer to, perhaps, a cosmetic surgery). Celebrities make their living by their appearance, and live according to a different set of rules than the average woman. Focus on love and kindness which come from your heart and make you look beautiful whatever you are.

4. **Don's try to do it fast. Give yourself time.** If you are working on losing weight, don't try to do it as quickly as possible. Listen to your body; it may be operating at a different time table. "Slow and steady wins the race" is the motto to follow when trying to stay in a better shape.

5. **Don't underestimate grooming yourself impeccably.** Taking the time to get dressed, style your hair, and groom yourself can ease your anxiety about the extra weight. Make self-care a priority: the dishes and laundry can wait. Put yourself first, so you can willingly – rather than resentfully – tackle household chores.

Having a positive body image of yourself is not about what you look like, but how you feel inside.

If you know that your body's changes are essential to your developing baby that gives you a reason to embrace these changes with love and smile.

Surrounding yourself with positive people gives you a boost of self-confidence.

During your pregnancy you can be more vulnerable to negative self-talk and it can affect you in a negative way. If you are feeling that you are not getting the support you need, share that with those around you.

A body massage or a makeover helps you to appreciate yourself and love your experiences.

A good massage or a makeover gives you a boost of joy and pleasant feelings about yourself. It is worth the investment as there is nothing more valuable than healing of the soul.

Go shopping for yourself!

What better excuse to go shopping. There are cute and even sophisticated maternity clothes to buy. This is your time to shine. Make the most of these wonderful 9 months.

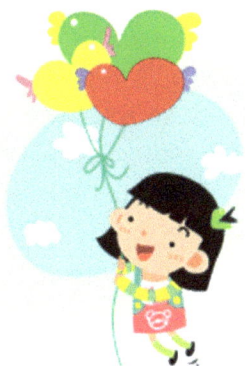

CHAPTER 17

Healthy Eating during Pregnancy. What and How to Eat during Pregnancy

Your food is the building material for your baby when you're pregnant. No wonder the old adage says 'a pregnant woman should eat for two'. But how true is this?

The answer is 'Yes, this is true' because healthy eating during pregnancy has a big effect on your health and the health of your baby. But it doesn't mean that you have to eat more food. What the saying actually means is eating more of the right kinds of foods and making sure that you are consuming just the right amount of nutrients to ensure a healthy baby as well as a healthy mother. Fail to feed your body properly during all nine months of your pregnancy and you both will suffer the nutritional consequences.

How much should you eat?

You don't need to double your food intake when you get pregnant. In fact, eating more than necessary is unwise and lead to excessive weight gain. On average, during the first trimester most women don't need any additional calories as the baby is tiny and doesn't need extra food to grow. But if you think you are a bit underweight you can add on 100 additional calories per day during the first trimester.

During the second and third trimester most women need about 300 additional calories per day as the baby is growing fast and need more nutrients to grow.

To find out how much calories you need to consume, first of all, you need to work out how many calories your body is burning each day when you're not pregnant. As a very general rule of thumb, you can refer to the table below:

Weight	Calories
50 kg	1680 Cal per day
60 kg	1800 Cal per day
70 kg	1920 Cal per day
80 kg	2040 Cal per day
90 kg	2155 Cal per day
100 kg	2270 Cal per day

Then, just add on 100 calories for the first trimester and 300 calories for the second and third trimester. This will be the amount of calories you need to consume during pregnancy.

How much food is 100 calories? How much extra food a day you can eat during the first trimester?

- one-third of a cheeseburger from McDonalds
- six pieces of California roll sushi
- five slices of turkey lunch meat
- 57 g of smoked salmon
- 57 g of cod, halibut or other white fish
- 85 g of boiled lobster or crab meat

- 1 jumbo size egg
- 1 slice of whole grain bread
- 2 slices of light bread
- one half of a taco
- 68 g of lean, roasted ham
- 1 cup of skim milk
- 1 cup of sweetened almond milk
- 1 cup of unsweetened soy milk
- 1 medium apple or large pear
- 1 medium orange or grapefruit
- 1 small size banana
- 1 cup of grapes

What kind of food you should eat when pregnant?

Your food should contain all the necessary vitamins, minerals and substances for developing a healthy baby. You should consume foods from all the food groups including dairy, grains, protein, carbohydrates and of course plenty of fresh fruits and vegetables.

The table below can be used as a general guide what food to eat during pregnancy and how much to eat. You should consume foods from different food groups every day. Great variety of food you eat ensures great variety of nutrients for you and the baby.

Food Group	Servings per day	Example of one servings
Meat, fish, poultry, eggs – protein foods.	3	3 medium whole eggs 110 g canned tuna or sardines 120 g canned salmon 120 g skinless chicken 120 g cooked turkey 120 g lean beef, lamb, veal or pork 130 g cooked shellfish 130 g (before cooking) fresh fish

Milk and dairy – calcium+protein foods.	4	1 cup (250 ml) of low-fat milk ⅓ cup non-fat dry milk ½ cup low-fat cottage cheese 200 g low-fat yoghurt 200 g low-fat frozen yoghurt ⅓ cup grated cheese ½ cup pasteurized ricotta cheese 250 mL (1 cup) custard
Fruits and vegetables (including green leafy and yellow vegetables and yellow fruits)	4-5	½ medium size grapefruit ½ cup grapefruit juice ½ cup orange juice ¼ cup lemon juice ½ medium-size mango ¼ medium-size papaya ⅓ cup strawberries ½ size kiwi fruit ¾ tomato juice 1 sweet potato or baking potato, baked in skin 1 medium-size tomato ⅔ cup blueberries or raspberries 2 large fresh apricots ½ medium-size mango ¼ medium-size papaya 1 large nectarine 1 small persimmon 1 cup coleslaw mix 1 packed cup green leafy lettuce, such as rocket, or red or green leaf ¼ cup cooked pumpkin ½ small sweet potato or yam 1 medium size apple ½ cup apple juice 1 medium size banana 2 small plums ½ cup fresh raw mushrooms

Fruits and vegetables (continued)	4-5	½ cup onion ½ Seaweed ½ cup Spinach and dark green leafy vegetables ½ cup cooked green beans
Whole grains, legumes, breads	6	1 cup cooked wholegrain cereal, such as rolled oats 2 cups air-popped popcorn ½ cup granola or muesli 1 cup cooked wholegrain cereal, such as rolled oats 2 tablespoons wheat germs ½ cup cooked millet, bulgur, couscous, polenta, barley or quinoa 2 cups air-popped popcorn 2 slices of bread 1 medium bread roll 1 cup cooked rice, pasta, noodles 1 cup porridge
Fat and oils	3-4 (depends on your weight gain)	1 tablespoon vegetable oil 2 tablespoons 'light' margarine 1 tablespoon regular mayonnaise 2 tablespoons regular salad dressing ¼ cup sour cream 2 tablespoons regular cream cheese 2 tablespoons peanut or almond butter
Fluids	At least 6-8 (250ml) glasses daily – 2 litres a day	Water Juices Milk, soups, decaffeinated coffee and tea are counted in the daily amount of fluids

Some nutrients are particularly important, so make sure to include them in your diet:

Calcium is necessary to keep your bones from getting depleted and to help your baby's bones develop. You need about 1,000 milligrams of calcium per day when you are pregnant or breast-feeding, which is going to be about 400 milligrams more than you need when you aren't pregnant or breastfeeding. Some examples of serving sizes for calcium-rich foods are:

Food Calcium

Yogurt 230 g – 415 mg
Cheese 43 g – 275 mg
Salmon 85 mg – 181 mg
Spinach 2 cups – 120 mg

Other sources of calcium include: broccoli, sardines, dark leafy greens like spinach, kale, turnips, and collard greens, fortified cereals, corn flakes, fortified orange juice, soybeans, fortified soy-milk enriched breads, grains, and waffles.

Iron is essential for the manufacture of red blood cells that carry oxygen around the body. During pregnancy iron is needed in larger amounts because the mother's blood volume increases and the baby's blood is also developing.

A lack of iron in your diet causes iron deficiency anaemia which is a risk factor for premature delivery, low birth weight and anaemia in the baby. Pregnant women need 27 milligrams (mg) of iron per day (non-pregnant women -18 mg per day).

Rich iron foods are:

Food Iron content

Beans 1 cup – 5 mg
Spinach 2 cups – 3 mg
Beef 100 g – 3 mg
Lamb 100 g – 2.5 mg

Turkey 100 g – 2.3 mg
Chicken 100 g – 1.2 mg
Salmon 100 g – 1.7 mg
Dried apricots ½ cup – 2.1 mg
Broccoli ½ cup – 0.6 mg

Iron is found in food in two forms, heme and non-heme iron. Heme iron, which makes up 40 percent of the iron in meat, poultry, and fish, is well absorbed. Non-heme iron, 60 percent of the iron in animal tissue and all the iron in plants (fruits, vegetables, grains, nuts) is less well absorbed.

You can get heme-iron by eating food such as red meats, fish, and poultry (basically, food from animal sources). Iron-rich plant (non-heme iron) foods include cooked beans, lentils, and enriched pasta. Many breakfast cereals are also iron-fortified.

Most doctors recommend that women take a daily iron supplement during the last trimester, but eating plenty of dark green vegetables (like broccoli and spinach), whole meal and strawberries throughout the entire pregnancy can all help to boost iron levels more naturally. Avoid drinking tea or coffee with iron products since it can interfere with the way the body absorbed iron either though supplementation or natural food intake.

Fatty Acids

The body's cells need linoleic acid and alpha-linoleic acid in order to reproduce. This is especially necessary during pregnancy when that cell production creates new life. Foods with high concentrates of these important fatty acids include salmon, herring, sardines and fresh-water trout. You can eat up to 340 g per week of these fish. You can eat up to 170g per week of albacore (white) tuna. It's OK to eat these fish because they don't contain a lot of mercury, a metal that can be harmful to a baby during pregnancy.

Other sources of fatty acids are: fish oil, soy, eggs, broccoli, and dark green vegetables.

You may have heard that flaxseed and flaxseed oils are good sources of omega-3 fatty acids. Some studies on animals have shown that flaxseed can be harmful during pregnancy. We don't know enough about the effects of flaxseed on human pregnancy. So it's best not to use flaxseed or flaxseed oil if you're pregnant or breastfeeding.

Folic Acid (B-Vitamins)

Every pregnant woman is told to eat foods rich in folic acid. Why? Folic acid plays an important role in the production of red blood cells and helps your baby's neural tube develop into her brain and spinal cord. Here's how much folic acid is recommended each day in terms of pregnancy:

While you're trying to conceive: 400 mcg
For the first three months of pregnancy: 400 mcg
For months four to nine of pregnancy: 600 mcg
While breastfeeding: 500 mcg

For an immediate boost in folic acid, consider adding more spinach, collard greens, kale, turnip greens and romaine lettuce into your daily diet. Just one large plate of these delicious leafy greens can provide you with almost all of your daily needs for folic acid. Other foods rich in folic acid include Asparagus, Broccoli, oranges, papaya, grapefruit, grapes, banana, cantaloupe and strawberries.

Beans and pulses especially high in folic acid include pinto beans, lima beans, green peas, black-eyed peas and kidney beans. A small bowl of any type of lentils will give you the majority of your recommended daily amounts for folate.

Avocado, okra, brussel sprouts, sunflower seeds, peanuts, nuts, beets and cauliflower are also contain lots of folic acid.

Zinc is necessary for the production, repair, and functioning of DNA – the body's genetic blueprint and a basic building block of cells. So getting enough zinc is particularly important for the rapid cell growth that occurs during pregnancy. Get your full share (about 15 mg a day) via a supplement or by eating turkey, beef, lamb, pork, chicken, almonds, beans, wheat germ, yogurt, oatmeal, corn, eggs, fortified breads and cereals, and cooked shellfish, especially oysters.

Manganese (about 2 mg a day) is important for good reproductive function — in other words, a baby-making essential. Spinach, carrots, broccoli, whole grains, nuts, bananas, and raisins are all good sources of manganese.

Iodine is another nutrient that is important for your baby's brain development. To ensure adequate iodine either: eat fish one to three times a week, (limit high mercury types) and/or use iodised salt or take a multivitamin for pregnancy that contains iodine.

Vitamin D is mostly made in the skin by the action of sunlight, but a small amount can come from foods like oily fish, egg yolks, margarine and some brands of milk. Vitamin D is important for the development of your baby's bones and teeth and low levels can cause muscle weakness and pain in women. You may be vitamin D deficient, if you: have darker skin, cover most of your body in clothing, spend most of your time indoors.

Do I need to take extra vitamins and supplements when pregnant?

This is the questions with many answers. It all depends on several things:

- Is your daily diet rich enough with good nutrients and vitamins?

- What is your personal attitude to artificial vitamins and supplements? Do you trust them?
- Do you know which nutrients and vitamins you need to replace?

If your diet is good and rich with all the vitamins and nutrients, then you don't need any artificial vitamins or supplements. (except of folic acid, which is vital for pregnancy).

If you think that you don't have enough of good nutrients in your diet, then taking multivitamins and supplements is definitely not a bad idea. Discuss this with your doctor or dietician. Just remember that there is no substitute for good diet and the nutrients from good food are the best nutrients.

Listen to your intuition when making this decision about the multivitamins. How do you personally feel about taking them? Do you personally need them or not? But, of course, look at your diet first, before making any decision.

Do I really need to count consumed calories when I am pregnant?

Counting calories is not necessary if you're generally healthy and don't have problems with eating. Instead, it is wise to step on the scale at least 1-2 times a week and check your weight. If you gain weight according schedule (about 500g per week on average) you consume the right amount of calories. Adjust your food intake according to your weight.

Remember to wait yourself at the same time, for example first thing in the morning, or just before going to bed. If you do it in different times of the day it is easy to get false results, as the wait varies during the day depending on eating, drinking, going to the toilet etc.

Like we said before during the first trimester most women don't need any additional calories per day. During the second and third trimester most women need 300 additional calories per day. But there are four important exceptions to this formula.

First, if you are overweight you will need fewer calories than per formula. Second, if you are seriously underweight, you will need much more calories to restore normal weight. Third, if you are a teenager, you may need extra additional calories also, as your body is still growing. Fourth, if you're pregnant with twins (or more babies) you will need to add on 300 additional calories per each baby per day.

To avoid confusion it is always the best to consult your doctor or nutritionist what to do in each particular situation.

Can vegetarian diet be healthy during pregnancy?

Vegetarian diet is safe during pregnancy if you get enough protein, calcium, minerals, folic acid and other vitamins with the food you eat.

Protein.

If you eat eggs and milk products, getting enough protein is not a problem. If you are a vegan you need to make sure that you eat enough protein rich vegetarian foods. During pregnancy it is recommended to consume around 70 grams of protein per day, which is only about 25 grams more than you need when you are not pregnant.

Sources of Vegetarian Proteins.

Food	Amount of 1 serving (20 grams of protein)
Firm tofu	1 cup
Soft tofu	1¼ cup
Peanuts	3 oz. (85g)

Cooked beans such as: chickpeas, kidney beans, baked beans, pinto beans, refried beans, lentils or black beans	1½ cups
Soy milk	three 8-oz. (225g) glasses
Wholemeal pasta	3.2 oz (90g) before cooking
Wheat germ	⅓ cup
Bran Oats	1 cup uncooked, 2 cups cooked
Nuts (walnuts, pecans or almonds)	3.2 oz. (90 g)
Sesame, pumpkin or sunflower seeds	2.1 oz. (60g)
Green garden peace	¾ cup
Tempeh	3.2 oz. (90g)
Miso	¼ cup
Wholegrain bread	4 slices
Peanuts	40g
Uncooked quinoa	½ cup

Calcium.

For an ovo-lacto vegetarian, maintaining a sufficient level of calcium in the body would not be a problem. If you are a vegan, you need to make sure that you consume calcium rich food from non-animal sources.

Calcium rich food for vegans.

Food	Amount per one serving
Sesame seeds	3 tablespoons
Cooked greens such as spinach or silverbeet	1 ½ cups
Chinese cabbage (bokchoy)	3 cups
Cooked edamame (soybeans in their shells)	1 ½ cups
Blackstrap molasses	2 ½ tablespoons

You need to consume about 4 servings of calcium food each day when you are pregnant.

Other sources of calcium rich foods can be: tofu, dried figs, almonds, rice milk fortified with calcium, dried beans and flaxseeds.

Vitamins

Vitamins deficiencies are rare in vegetarians but vegans often don't get enough of vitamin B^{12}. If you are a vegan make sure to take supplements which contain B^{12} as well as folic acid and iron.

Other sources of B^{12} include B^{12} fortified cereal, soy milk, yeast, and fortified meat substitutes.

Don't forget about vitamin D which is produced by your skin when you're on the sun. Food sources of vitamin D are fatty fish, eggs, margarine, fortified juices, soy milk, fortified breads and fortified cereals.

What if you're lactose intolerant.

Milk and dairy products are great sources of calcium and proteins. Your growing baby must have enough of these vital nutrients for its healthy development. Make sure that your diet is full of other non-dairy foods which contain calcium and proteins.

Try to experiment taking hard cheeses and yogurts. You may discover that during the second and third trimester your digestive system can handle them normally.

You can also use lactose-free milk, calcium fortified drinks (like soy milk, juices etc), take lactase tablets before consuming milk or milk-products, or use other calcium or protein alternative.

I am addicted to junk food. What should I do?

Some people complaint that they can't resist chips, doughnuts, sweets, biscuits, pastries, sugary drinks, chocolate, ice-cream and other junky foods. They say it makes them feel good.

The main problem is that these foods are nutritionally empty, addictive, give you 'bad' extra calories and in a long run can poison your body with toxins. These better to be avoided during pregnancy.

It is better to replace them with fresh and dried fruits, nuts, wholegrain baked goods, muesli bars, yogurts and smoothies, cheeses and bread sticks. Use water and fresh juices instead of drinking sugary soft drinks.

Breaking 'junk food habit' can be difficult at first but there are some ways that make the withdrawal painless and even enjoyable:

- Plan all your meals and snacks in advance. Everyday take time to make a plan what you are going to eat to breakfast, lunch, dinner and use for snacks between the main meals. Make healthy choices when you plan and follow these instead of grabbing something at the nearest fast food place.
- Don't provoke your temptation by keeping no junk food in the house. When you go to shop buy plenty of fresh and dry fruits, vegetables, nuts and other natural snacks. Don't buy sweets, biscuits, chocolates, chips and other junk food when shopping for food. (Note: small to moderate amount

of chocolate is proven to be good in pregnancy. According to the new research, chocolate during pregnancy positively affect baby's emotional heath.)

- Make healthy substitutions. An ice cream replace with a cup of sweet fruit smoothie, a biscuits with a healthy muesli bar, sweets with dry fruits snacks, seeds or nuts etc.

- When you eat - think of the baby. All the food you put inside your stomach goes to your baby. Many women find that thinking of their babies make them stop eating junk food. No mom deliberately wants to feed her child with junk before he/she is born! To make you remember more of your baby, you can surround yourself with the pictures of beautiful babies: put them in your wallet, on your desk, in your handbag and etc. These pictures will remind you that you are eating for two.

- Set your limits. Eating small amount of junk food once in a while is OK during pregnancy, but only if you are able to control yourself and don't slip into a binge. If eating a single doughnut, a few biscuits or other sweets brings lots of pleasure, than do it once or twice a week but always remember to know your limits.

Eating out for two.

When you eat out during pregnancy always remember that not all restaurants are good during pregnancy. You wouldn't chose something likesushi bar restaurant with limited cooked choices or spicy food restaurant that make you nauseous more than usual.

Go for a green salad, vegetables soup, whole grained breads and protein meals like fish, seafood, chicken or lean meat. Your food is better to be grilled, steamed, barbecued, and/or poached. Avoid deep fried and fatty foods. Ask for fruity desert instead of creamy and sugary one.

What foods you should avoid during pregnancy?

Some foods are not safe during pregnancy because they often carry bacteria which can cause severe food poisoning. It is better to avoid these kinds of foods while you're pregnant. These foods are:

- Soft and semi-soft cheese unless it is fully cooked and served hot. This includes ricotta, fetta, camembert, brie and blue cheeses.
- Unpasteurised milk and dairy products made with unpasteurised milk.
- Soft serve ice-cream and also homemade icecream or gelatiicecream (especially those that have been made with raw eggs.
- Raw or undercooked eggs. Cook eggs until the yolk and white are hard.
- Chocolate mousse and fresh mayonnaise in delis, restaurants or in someone's home which may contain raw egg.
- Meat with pink or red bits (not properly cooked), especially if it's cooked on a barbecue, or as part of a ready meal.
- All paté should be avoided, whether made from meat, fish or vegetables.
- Cured meat products, such as prosciutto and salami, also carry a risk and are best avoided.
- Chicken that is cooked and served cold, such as in a salad or sandwich bar.
- Shark (Flake), Swordfish, Broadbill or Marlin because thee contain mercury.
- Avoid fish in sushi as it is usually raw and not safe during pregnancy.
- Raw oysters, shellfish and prawns.
- Bean sprouts carry a risk of salmonella including snow pea sprouts, mung beans, alfalfa sprouts and sunflower sprouts.

- Alcohol drinks should be completely avoided. It is a toxin which cross the placenta and affect your baby.
- Caffeine drinks should be limited during pregnancy. It is generally recommended that 200 mg of caffeine a day is safe which amounts to about two mugs of instant coffee, four cups of medium-strength tea or 6 cups of cola. Coffee from a café can amount to more than 200 mg in one cup, depending on how it's made.

Artificial sweeteners (sugar substitutes) during pregnancy.

If you're trying to reduce the sugar and calories in your diet, you may be turning to artificial sweeteners or other sugar substitutes. Many women do the same.

Today artificial sweeteners and other sugar substitutes are found in a variety of food and beverages marketed as "sugar-free" or "diet," including soft drinks, chewing gum, jellies, baked goods, candy, fruit juice, and ice cream and yogurt.

Most artificial sweeteners are probably safe during pregnancy but some research is still inconclusive. Here is the list of sugar substitutes that are commonly used today.

Sucralose (Splenda): It's sugar, sort of. At least it starts out life that way, before being chemically processed into a form that your body won't be able to absorb, making it sweet revenge (it's calorie-free). It has been approved by the FDA for pregnant women to consume — so sweeten your day (and your coffee, tea, yogurt) with it if you want. It's also stable for cooking and baking (unlike aspartame). Still, consume it in moderation as moderation is the key to all diets.

Aspartame (Equal, NutraSweet): Many experts think it's harmless, others think it's an unsafe artificial sweetener, pregnant or not. A packet or two of aspartame every now and then probably will not do any harm. Just avoid consuming aspartame during pregnancy in large amounts and steer clear of it altogether if PKU is on your medical chart.

Saccharin (Sweet'N Low): Well, the FDA has deemed saccharin as a safe sweetener, but there have been some questionable studies, so it is your choice if you're going to worry about them or not. One advice to follow: don't consume it too much.

Acesulfame-K (Sunnette): This substitute is also FDA-approved and has 200 times the sweetness of regular sugar. You'll find it in baked goods, gelatin, gum, and soft drinks, but again — moderation is key.

Sorbitol: Sorbitol is actually a nutritive sweetener, which is fine for women during pregnancy. But while it can't hurt your baby, it can have unpleasant gastro effects on you: in large doses, it can cause stomach upset and diarrhoea, something no pregnant woman wants to have. It's safe in moderate amounts but can lead to excess pregnancy weight gain if you overdo it. Sorbitol has more calories than other substitutes and less sweetness than regular sugar.

Mannitol: Like sorbitol, it's a nutritive sweetener that's safe for pregnant women, and moderate amounts are fine, but its poor absorption by your body means it can cause unfortunate goings-on in your stomach.

Xylitol: A sugar alcohol derived from plants (it's naturally occurring in many fruits and veggies), xylitol can be found in chewing gum, toothpaste, candies, and some foods. Considered safe during pregnancy in moderate amounts.

Stevia: The latest sugar substitute to hit the market, this sweetener is derived from a South American shrub. Stevia hasn't been approved by the FDA as a sweetener (it's considered a dietary supplement), and no clear research proves it's safe during pregnancy. Your best bet is to check with your practitioner before using it.

Lactose: Avoid this milk sugar if you're lactose intolerant, but otherwise, it's safe during pregnancy.

Best Pregnancy Foods.

You know you should always eat healthy; especially now when you're expecting, you are trying to feed yourself just the best foods. But there are so much conflicting information floating around. Many people say that fish is the best food but others say it contains too much mercury. The same conflicting stories go for meat, eggs and cheese during pregnancy.

So what should you eat which is safe and is really the best for pregnancy?

Don't worry...There are lots of ways to ensure that you and your baby are getting the nutrients you both need. There are many foods that can provide all you need. Here you can read about some of the super foods of pregnancy. You don't need to eat all these foods, just choose your favorites and enjoy them.

Avocados: a real super food, especially for pregnancy time! Avocados are full with folate (vital to forming your baby's brain and nervous system), potassium, vitamin C and vitamin B6 (which not only helps baby's tissue and brain growth, but may also help with your morning sickness), potassium (which is good for your heart, muscles and nerves), anti-oxidants (helps you to maintain strengths by improving your immune system) and many more other nutrients.

Avocados are good in salads; as a spread on your whole-grain roll as a healthy substitute for mayo. Keep in mind that avocados are high in fat (though the very good kind), so don't overuse them if you're gaining too much weight.

Broccoli: another super food veggie which is packed with vitamins A and C, calcium and folic acid. It is a potent immune stimulant and a metabolism booster. Good as an addition into pasta or casseroles, stir-fry with fish or chicken, serve steamed (with or without a vinaigrette), or dunk in dip.

Carrots: This vegetable is full of variety of vitamins: vitamin A (so important for the development of your baby's bones, teeth and eyes), vitamins B6, vitamin C, folate and fibre. Carrots are perfect for munching on the go, in salads and as addition to many foods from sandwiches to cakes to muffins.

Eggs: For meat eaters and vegetarians (unless you're a vegan) an egg is a great source of protein (a great brain's building material), DHA and choline (a nutrient that plays a big role in boosting your baby's brain cells), omega-3 fatty acid and lutein and zeaxanthin (which are antioxidants found in egg yolks and are good for the eye sight). Eggs can be cooked in many different ways: boiled, fried or scrambled. Add them to your salads and sandwiches. But be careful about raw eggs: they can contain dangerous bacteria Salmonella. Your daily intake will depend on a number of factors, including health history, nutritional status (what else you eat) and activity level. Ask your practitioner how many eggs to eat per day (or per week) in your particular situation.

Soy beans: these are also considered to be a super food as they are packed with protein, calcium, folic acid and vitamins A and B. Everything that you and baby need! You can eat soy beans as a snack (salt them lightly, and you'll never miss the chips), or tossed into just about anything you're cooking, from soups, to pasta, to casseroles, to chili, to stir-fry.

Lentils: are some of the most nutritious, and at the same time economical, foods in the world. Lentils are rich sources of protein, folic acid, dietary fiber, vitamin C, B vitamins, essential amino acids and trace minerals. A 100 g serving of lentils contains 60 g carbohydrates, 31 g dietary fiber, 1 g fat, 26 g protein, 0.87 mg thiamine, 479 µg of folate and 7.5 mg iron. Among the winter growing legumes, lentils have the highest concentration of antioxidants.

Mangoes: Mangoes contain more vitamins A and C for a delicious bite than a salad. It also contains lots of potassium, copper, vitamin-B6 (pyridoxine), and vitamin-E. Blend it into smoothies or soups, chop it up in salsas or relishes, simply scoop and enjoy.

Nuts: Nuts are a great source of important minerals such as copper, manganese, magnesium, selenium, zinc, potassium, calcium and vitamin E. And even though they're high in fat, it's mainly the good-for-you kind – especially baby-brain-boosting DHA, which is found in walnuts. Eat the as a snack and toss them into salads, pasta, meat or fish dishes, and baked goods.

Porridge: They're good for your stomach; can reduce the puffiness from your feet, hands and face. They're full of fibre, B vitamins, and iron and a lots of other minerals. Different grains can be used: oats, rice, wheat, barley, corn and legumes. Fill your breakfast bowl with them and enjoy your delicious meal.

Spinach: Fresh leaves are rich source of several vital anti-oxidant vitamins like vitamin A, vitamin C, and flavonoid poly phenolic antioxidants such as lutein, zea-xanthin and beta-carotene, folate, iron, vitamin A, vitamin K and calcium. Eat it raw, in a salad (especially one with almonds and mandarin oranges), or as a wilted bed for fish or chicken, or layered in lasagne.

Yoghurt: It contains beneficial bacteria (probiotics) that help keep your digestive and immune systems humming, your arteries flexible, and your triglyceride levels and blood pressure low – essentials for healthy pregnancy functioning. Yogurt contains as much calcium as milk – but it's packed with protein and folate too. Blend it with fruit into satisfying smoothies, layer with muesli in a breakfast parfait, use it as a low-calorie substitute for sour cream or mayo in sandwich fillings, dips and salad dressings, or simply spoon it out of the pot.

Whole meal bread is a long-term energy provider and full of fibre. It contains some calcium, iron, B vitamins and folic acid.

Apples: The old adage is saying 'An apple a day keep doctors away'. It's absolutely true as apples is notable for its impressive list of phtyto-nutrients, and anti-oxidantsas. Apples contain good quantities of vitamin-C and beta-carotene, lots of fibre (good for the bowel), minerals such as potassium, phosphorus, and calcium. Apples have everything to keep you healthy during this important time of expecting.

Red pepper: A super-source of vitamins A and C, with plenty of B6 in the bargain, a red pepper is one of nature's sweetest ways to eat your vegetables. Chop them into salsa, slice them into stir-fries and pasta dishes, or roast or grill them (with a little olive oil, garlic and lemon) and serve them up in sandwiches, salads or antipastos.

Dark green, leafy, fresh or frozen vegetables are packed with vitamin C, fibre and folic acid.

Potatoes: This food is a main source of carbohydrate which gives long-term energy. They are packed with fibre, some iron and some vitamins. Great when baked, boiled, puree, in salads or soups. Note: potatoes chips are not healthy. This way of cooking kills all the goods in this otherwise great product.

Lean red meat and poultry contain protein, iron and some vitamins and minerals. It helps to cook them with little or no fat, oil or salt.

Dried fruit such as apricots is full of iron, fibre, vitamin C and other vitamins, as well as minerals.

Fish is a great source of protein – low in fat and high in iron. Try to include two portions a week of omega-3 rich fish such as tuna, trout, salmon or sardines.

Whole meal pasta and brown rice both provide long-term energy as well as lots of fibre.

Berries are a great and tasty food for pregnancy. Blueberries, raspberries, strawberries and blackberries are delicious snacks and taste great in pancakes and on top of cereal. Berries are packed with vitamin C, potassium, folate, and fiber. Berries contain high levels of antioxidants that protect cells from damage by harmful free radicals.

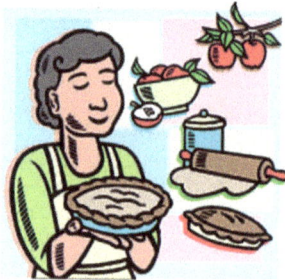

Regarding any pregnancy food you eat follow this eternal principle:

"Let food be thy medicine and medicine be thy food"
                                                        – Hippocrates

CHAPTER 18

Sex during Pregnancy

t is common for couples to wonder whether sex is safe when they discover they are pregnant. There is no evidence that sex (coitus or masturbation), whether leading to orgasm or not, has any damaging effect on a baby. Sex is safe during pregnancy. The baby is protected by the amniotic fluid in the womb, by your abdomen and by the mucus plug which seals your cervix and helps guard against infections.

In fact, sex is good during pregnancy as it promotes bonding between partners, relaxes you, makes you feel good and eliminates stress. It can also be beneficial for a positive body image during pregnancy.

There are some important circumstances, however, in which you may be advised not to have intercourse. These situations are:

- You have a history of miscarriage
- If your water has broken
- History of premature birth or labour
- If you have placenta previa, or a very low-lying placenta
- If you have an incompetent cervix or if it has dilated.
- If you or your partner has a sexually transmitted disease.
- If you experience unexplained vaginal bleeding or discharge.

Will sex feel as good?

For some women it feels even better, but for some are not. Some people don't feel any difference whether pregnant or not. However, many women experience decreased sexual desire, especially in the early pregnancy and after the 30th week. The reasons for this decline in libido are many: hormonal surges, early and late pregnancy complaints, discomforts, increased vulnerability and sensitivity during early and late stages of pregnancy. .

During the middle phase of pregnancy (from about 12-14 weeks until about 28 to 30 weeks), many women find they have a renewed interest in sex, as they feel physically better and more energetic: morning sickness has passed and the belly is not very big yet. There are now fewer concerns about miscarriage and both partners have usually come to accept the pregnancy, if there was initial ambivalence. Women often feel more relaxed now, with sexual arousal and sensuality often becomes heightened.

Accepting and loving your own feelings about sex during pregnancy is the way to approach this sensitive issue. Accept that everything you experience is normal: increased or decreased sexual desire, uncomfortable feelings or feelings more sexual than ever, feeling cautious about sex or loving it. All these feelings are individual and different for every woman and every pregnancy. This is all normal. Just love and appreciate them.

Will your partner's sex drive change?

Most people find their pregnant partner truly attractive. But some partners may worry about the women's health and fear that sex can hurt the baby or even self-consciousness about making love in the presence of their unborn child. Advice is here to focus more on intimacy, nurturing and caring about each others feelings more and more especially when pregnancy progresses.

The best sex positions during pregnancy.

Many people look at sex position in pregnancy as the right one and the wrong one. And many people have this idea that there is one right (or safe) way to have sex during pregnancy.

But the truth is that a good sex position for pregnant sex is one where:

- Both partners are physically comfortable.
- The position allows for the kind of sex and physical contact you want to have.

Great sex requires a flexibility of thoughts and a willingness to try new things when the old ones aren't working anymore (for example, the missionary position with you on the bottom and your partner on top may become increasingly awkward as your pregnant belly begins to grow).

So, here are some time-tested positions and tips for making love while you're pregnant:

Woman on Top

This classic "cowgirl" position is a great move as it takes all the pressure off of your abdomen and allows you to control the depth and frequency of thrusting. It also gives your partner a great view!

Woman on Back

This position is like the missionary position only without any added pressure to your abdomen or uterus. You lie on your back and raise your knees up towards your chest. Your partner then kneels between your legs and enters from the front. You can even rest your feet on your partner's chest for support. Place a pillow under your bottom for added comfort. This position isn't recommended after the fourth month – you should avoid lying on your back for extended periods after this point in your pregnancy, as the weight of your uterus could block blood vessels that supply your uterus and legs.

Side-lying positions.

This position has you and your partner lying on your sides facing one another. It keeps weight off of your abdomen while supporting your uterus at the same time. It is also very intimate, as you and your partner are both facing each other.

Spooning

Spooning is a great position to use during the late stages of pregnancy. Both you and your partner lie on your sides, with your partner behind you, facing your back. Entry is from the rear. This position is very comfortable for pregnant women because it keeps the weight off your belly and allows for only shallow penetration. Sometimes, deep penetration is very uncomfortable in the late stages of pregnancy.

Sitting

Get your partner to sit on the edge of the bed or in a chair and then straddle him. This will keep any added pressure off of your stomach, and allows for a very intimate experience.

Rear Entry

"Doggy style" position is a favourite of many pregnant women. This is because it allows for deeper penetration and also gives you the opportunity to support your stomach and breasts. You get on all fours and, using pillows, support your stomach and chest. Your partner then stands or kneels behind you, and enters from behind. Because deep thrusting is involved, be sure to tell your partner exactly what feels good for you.

What about oral sex?

Oral sex is OK. It is safe for you and your baby and it is considered as a good solution if intercourse seems too risky. Don't do it if you or your partner has sexual transmitted infections or herpes infection which affect lips or genitals.

Have faith - where there's a will, there's a way. With a little experimenting, you and your partner are sure to find a technique that works for you.

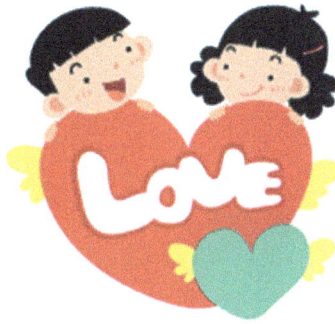

CHAPTER 19

Quitting Bad Habits – Establishing Good Habits

Smoking, drinking, overeating, taking drugs, eating junk food or extreme dieting, not getting enough sleep, too little or too much exercise – all these bad habits can affect the health of pregnant women and their babies.

We all know that bad habits are very tough to break. But if you're pregnant, it's time to put your baby's health and well-being above your own indulgence. Now is the time to implement a new lifestyle, break a few habits and start your journey towards a healthier you.

Remember, your baby's health depends on what you do, what you eat and what you use. So go ahead and break these bad habits that seem to plague the women of today.

Alcohol. There is no safe amount of alcohol you can drink during pregnancy. It used to be believed that drinking moderate amounts (a drink a day) was relatively safe. But it's only recently been discovered that children of women who drank during pregnancy — even those who had as little as one drink a day — were experiencing developmental problems throughout their childhood and even into adolescence.

For the unborn child, the alcohol interferes with his ability to get enough oxygen and nourishment for normal cell development in the brain and other body organs.

Even a small amount of alcohol can cause permanent damage to the child. The best advice here is not to drink during pregnancy at all, not even a small amount and stop drinking if you've been drinking. Don't worry too much if you had a few occasional drinks before realizing you shouldn't have had it. It will be OK if you don't drink anymore and start on a healthy life style for the rest of your pregnancy.

What are the consequences of alcohol drinking during pregnancy?

If mothers drink during pregnancy, various amounts of damage can occur to their children:

- Children may show slow growth and developmental delay, unusual facial features, irritability, brain and neurological disorders, mental retardation and problems with their attachment to their parents.
- Older children may have problems with learning, low tolerance for frustration, inadequate social boundaries and difficulty reading.
- Teenagers can have continuous learning problems, depression, anxiety and inappropriate sexual behaviour.

Many children from drinking mothers are born with 'foetal alcohol syndrome' (FAS). FAS is characterized by:

- Facial deformities.
- Slow and retarded development.
- Brain and neurological problems

Children with FAS are small, underweight and very weak. As they get older, they often have trouble with learning, attention, memory and problem solving. They may have poor coordination, be impulsive and have speech and hearing problems. They can't cope with stress, have low adaptability to new situations, and suffer from anxiety and unexplainable mood swings.

FAS does not go away. Its effects last a lifetime. Adults with FAS often have trouble with work and personal relationships. Many also have legal problems and get involved in crimes, drug and alcohol problems, have high risk of becoming homeless.

This problem cannot be cured. Children who are born with FAS will need regular medical care, hearing aids and/or eyeglasses. They will also need special help at school and often need special services and support to help them live on their own.

Tips for quitting alcohol:

1. Be aware of your vulnerabilities.
   Be aware of situations in which you will be susceptible to the temptations of alcohol. It can be drinking parties where you drink because of the peer pressure or business functions where alcohol served freely or the other places where you feel you need to drink. Recognise that these places are not for pregnant women to attend, especially for those who are trying to quit drinking. Have excuses ready in order to avoid social gatherings focused around drinking.

2. Think of the reason why you want to stop drinking.
   The role of mother begins as soon as the child is conceived. No mother wants for her child to be sick and unhealthy. So your main reason to stop drinking is to protect your child from alcohol damage. Read everything about "fetal alcohol syndrome" and what consequences it has on a child's life. This knowledge will help you to abstain from alcohol drinking.

3. Choose the right people to be around with.

   Drunks have the ability to bring others down and make them drink. It is better for you and your baby to stay away from such people. If you have a group of drinking buddies, pregnancy is a time to find other ways to bond or cut them off completely. You may have to accept losing a few "friends".

4. Don't keep any alcohol at home.

   Keeping alcohol at home provoke your temptation to drink. Throw out all the bottles of alcohol from your cupboards, fridge and other places where you use to keep alcohol.

5. Seek help.

   Quitting on your own can be challenging. There are plenty of help available in form of support groups, psychological and cancelling services, spiritual groups and individuals who used to drink but now is willing to help others to stop drinking.

6. Mediate regularly.

   Meditation helps to control drinking urges by calming the mind and making your brain non-reactive. Meditation helps you to become mindful – the state when you are able to pay attention on purpose and direct your awareness on something you want to achieve (stay sober and healthy).

7. Find a nurturing spiritual path.

   Spirituality and faith can help you to get the strength and power to stop drinking alcohol. Your spiritual path is not necessarily what your friends and family follow. You should find something that moves you, that you feel intuitively resonate with. People may link Spirit with God, the Universe, the Light, Allah or the nature. It could be spiritual for them but if you can't feel their heart, all that means nothing to you. Begin exploring your personal spiritual path from reading classical books like "Varieties of Religious Experience' of William James and "The Art of Happiness" of Dalai Lama.

8. Get a Busy Life.

   Make yourself busy with good positive things that need to be accomplished before the birth of your baby. It can be something you love to do (like a hobby) or classes to improve health or parenting classes or a new course. Fill your life with purpose and desire to be good and helpful to others. This will make it easier for you to abstain from alcohol.

9. Exercise

   Physical activity will help you to stay in your best physical shape possible during the pregnancy. It will help your body resist cravings.

10. Eat healthy and drink plenty of water.

    Eating healthy is beneficial for you and your baby. It will also keep you feeling good and subsequently lower your desire to drink. Good hydration of the body does the same.

11. Reward your effort.

    At first it would be difficult for you not to drink alcohol. Accept that and find a way to reward yourself for the effort you put into this difficult but very positive task. In the end of each week of abstaining from alcohol you may reward yourself with a cute piece of jewellery or something else you like. This will make you feel appreciated and loved.

Smoking. When a pregnant woman smokes - the baby suffers. Every time a pregnant mother takes a drag from a cigarette, normal foetal breathing movements (a sign of a healthy foetus) are reduced within five minutes. Smoking places stress on the baby's heart and affects the development of its lungs. It makes it harder for your baby to get the oxygen and nourishment it needs. Other common problems associated with smoking during pregnancy are:

- Ectopic pregnancy and spontaneous abortion
- Premature rupture of membranes
- The placenta separating from the uterus
- Abnormal location of the placenta, which can cause massive bleeding during delivery and pre-term delivery.

Infants that are born to women who smoke during pregnancy have lower than average birth weight and are more likely to be small for their age. Low birth weight is associated with increased risk for death from sudden infant death syndrome.

Another study shows that children exposed to tobacco smoke in the womb are more likely to get asthma and different allergies.

Common question: "Can giving up smoking by going cold turkey hurt me or my baby?"

In fact, it is not only safe, but it's one of the best things you can do for yourself and your baby while you're pregnant. As soon as you stop smoking, your baby will start getting more oxygen, and the risk of miscarriage, premature labour, and other complications will fall.

Healthy Tips to Quit Smoking.

1. Write down all the reasons why you want to quit smoking. In fact it is the best if you write them down daily or at least revise them daily. The more you focus on the reasons to quit the more motivated you become.

2. Revise the situations where you most tempted to smoke and try to avoid them if possible.
3. Throw out all cigarettes, ashtrays and lighters and anything else that might remind you of smoking. Wash your clothes and clean your car to remove the smell of smoke.
4. Get support from family, friends and co-workers by letting them know that you're going to quit smoking.
5. Remember 4Ds principal: delay, deep breath, drink water and do something else.

Delay: the more you delay taking a cigarette the easier it becomes. The worst cravings normally last for a short time only. If you overcome this time, then the cravings subside.

Deep breathe: this should help you relax and centre yourself which eases (even stops) the cravings.

Drink water: it is a good idea to drink plenty of fluids to help flush the nicotine and other toxins out of your system.

Do something else: distract yourself from thinking of having a cigarette by going for a walk, watching a movie or visit a supportive friend. Try eating an apple or cleaning your teeth when you would normally have a cigarette. You could hold something else, such as a pen or beads, to replace the need to hold a cigarette, or chew some gum or eat or drink a healthy snack to have something other than a cigarette in your mouth.

6. Meditate daily. Meditation helps your mind to become less reactive to internal or external stimuli and helps to stop cravings completely.
7. Exercise daily. Exercising helps your body to produce endorphins (hormones of happiness) which make you feel happy and relaxed. This alone can eliminate the urge to smoke cigarettes.

Overeating.

If you are overweight, it is more likely that you overeat (although many overweight people would deny overeating).

How to know if you are overeating?

In general, people are overeating if they are gaining excessive amounts of weight. If you are taking in more calories than you need, you will gain weight. Most pregnant women need only about 2, 500 -2, 600 daily calories to meet their energy requirements. That's just 300 calories more than your normal requirements, depending on your height and activity.

You can start counting your daily calories to see how much you overeat and when.

Overeating during pregnancy increases your risk of:

- Developing gestational diabetes.
- Increased blood pressure.
- Painful and complicated labour.
- Increased chance for Caesarean delivery.
- Having an overweight baby which creates many health problems for the child not only at the time of delivery but in the future.

Tips to stop overeating when pregnant:

- Practice mindful awareness (or mindfulness) which helps to reduce cravings for more food or junk food and also make you constantly aware of your food choices and how much you actually eat.
- Meditate before you eat. Mediation will make you more aware of your feelings and you can derive more pleasure from your food, give the meal your full attention, and notice when you've had enough.
- Eat slowly and chew every bite.

- Make your food beautiful. Paying attention to the presentation of a meal can increase your awareness of the food in front of you and help you stop eating when you are comfortable.
- Choose low calories but high in volume foods.

Not getting enough sleep. Lack of sleep during pregnancy may put you at a higher risk for preterm birth, create stress, affect your moods and compromise your immune system. So when pregnant, make sure you have enough good sleep. No more working overtime, staying in office till late and ignoring your body's scream for a peaceful night of sleep.

Learn to take 20 minutes naps during the day. Learn to meditate or do yoga which is beneficial for the health of your nervous system and relaxation.

Tips for getting enough sleep:

- Make a strict sleep routine. Always go to bed at same time.
- Create a nice bed time ritual. This 'bed time' ritual can be: meditation, taking a warm bath, lighting candles, aromatherapy, light reading, listening to relaxing music.
- Don't eat heavy food late at night. Don't go to bed either hungry or stuffed. Don't take any stimulants such as nicotine, caffeine and alcohol.
- Create a nice peaceful atmosphere in your bedroom.
- Make your bed comfortable.
- Avoid any sleeping pills.
- Meditate and exercise daily.

Too little or too much exercise.

Exercise helps fight fatigue, excess weight, chances of diabetes and stroke and gives your metabolism a boost. However, too much exercise can be bad for you. Excessive exercising causes a lot of fat burn, which can interfere with your hormonal system. Similarly, too little exercise can make you obese, prone to

Diabetes Type 2 and negatively affect your ability to conceive due to hormonal fluctuations. So ideally aim for a 30 to 40 minute workout 5-7 times a week.

The biggest problem people have when quitting bad habits and establishing new ones that they start and then stop too quickly. Their motivation weakens in a few days and they slip back into old behavioral pattern.

The best way to quit bad habits is to replace them with good positive ones. If you just try to quit – you will create emptiness in your mind and soul. This emptiness must be filled with good and positive things (good habits). For example, when you got cravings for cigarettes, instead of having one, you try to shift your focus by doing something positive: meditation, walking, jogging, doing a yoga pose or etc.

Learning something new creates new neuronal pathways in the brain. These can replace old neuronal pathways which are responsible for an old negative habit. For example, learning to meditate can replace the habit of smoking cigarettes or drinking or overeating if you do your meditation regularly.

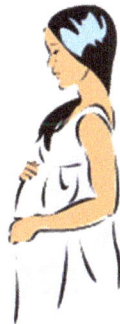

Motivation is what gets you started.
Habit is what keeps you going.

– Jim Ryun

Chapter 20

Two to Tango

The Father's Role during Pregnancy.

When a Father-to-be is told that much of his role will involve dispensing "emotional support", some men will have a job stopping their eyes glazing over! "Emotional" support and "moral" support are phrases that are often used as euphemisms, in situations where a person is effectively being told that they really have no role, or that there is nothing they can do. For example, in an episode of The Simpsons, a crisis hits the Springfield Power Plant. In this critical situation, where all hands are needed, Homer is told that his role will be to provide "moral support". In other words, "stay out of the way!"

But there can be no overstating how crucial the emotional support provided by a father is during the pregnancy process. Whether the pregnancy is unexpected or long-planned, there will be plenty of ups and downs before junior makes an appearance. And when these happen, it is important that you are there to lift your partner when they are down, to help her when she needs it and to make the entire experience as placid as possible.

The role of the father-to-be has also changed in modern times, so that it now includes much more hands-on, practical help and support. Breathing exercises, massage techniques and plenty to do around the home...providing emotional support has a much more physical dimension to it that you may have thought!

Your partner will face quite a journey in which you will share. From morning sickness to hormonal swings, many physical and emotional changes will take place during pregnancy. It is your patience, support and sympathy that will make the bad moments bearable and the high points memorable. And the more you grow into this supportive role, the more the bond between you, mother and baby will grow. Even before birth!

Whichever way the rollercoaster of pregnancy pans out for you and your partner, you get to share in a unique experience. And with that, you are being provided with a golden opportunity to build a greater bond with your partner. Building intimacy between you and your partner is a must during the pregnancy process and it is something that will reward your bond with her and with baby.

Remember, you too will face your own anxieties and doubts. There isn't a dad in the world who hasn't felt this way! But, by learning to recognise and cope with your own fears and flaws, you are preparing yourself for the life's greatest challenge and most rewarding gift. Parenthood.

And remember, you'll do great if you remember one thing:

Being a great father starts by being a great father-to-be. To be a great father-to-be, become the very definition of emotional support.

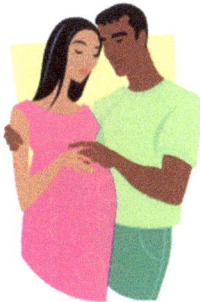

Helping mother to cope up with symptoms of pregnancy.

Morning Sickness

Morning sickness is caused by fluctuating hormone levels and is often one of the first signs of pregnancy. In reality, many men get caught out by the misnomer of "Morning" sickness; whilst it is most prevalent in the morning, morning sickness can strike at any time of day. Your sympathy for your partner shouldn't end at 12 noon!

Morning Sickness doesn't end at 12 Noon!

More than half of pregnant women will experience morning sickness in the first trimester, marked by bouts of nausea and vomiting. Typically these symptoms last from the 6th week of pregnancy until around the 12th week. However, some women will still experience bouts of morning sickness beyond the 12th week, with a small minority of women even experiencing morning sickness in the last trimester.

Morning sickness can come on quite suddenly and certain smells and odours can trigger it. Whilst some of these might be obvious, more everyday smells and odours may also be found to be problematic for your partner. These can be deodorants, cheeses or anything with a strong, distinct smell. Sometimes even the sight of certain foods that have a strong smell or taste associated with it can trigger nausea or vomiting. If this is the case, it is important not to see these aversions as being in any way trivial. Morning sickness can be very debilitating, so if certain foods or products are causing it, just get rid of them.

Remove anything that triggers morning sickness. If in doubt, chuck it out!

Remember that whilst you can't do anything to take away the morning sickness, you can do a great deal to mitigate the effects and make the experience much more bearable by being sympathetic, supportive and helpful.

Here are some practical tips:

You fill up the car. Your partner may feel overwhelmed by powerful odours. This can result in spontaneous bouts of sickness. Be aware of this possibility and account for it. Expand on this by thinking of other possible situations where you can prevent unnecessary bouts of sickness.

If you own deodorant or aftershaves that trigger her morning sickness, don't wear them. In fact, store them away or bin them completely.

If your partner is spending extended periods in the bathroom, support her by staying with her. Bring her iced water or hold back her hair. You don't have to be there, but by showing her that you want to be there, you are making a small but very positive sacrifice for your relationship. This will also convey to your partner a sense that you will be a better and more involved father.

Encourage your partner to eat small, balanced meals regularly. 3 meals a day really isn't an option during this phase. You should take a proactive role in this by cooking for her. Avoid big portions and ensure that meals are nutritious and do not contain foodstuffs that may cause more morning sickness.

Don't joke about it. The most likely result of that will be to drive a wedge between the two of you and negate all the other good work you are doing.

Cravings

Fathers-to-be will likely already be aware of food cravings; they are a facet of pregnancy that extends into popular culture. In fact, we all probably know more than one man who's first question to a pregnant woman won't be "Is it a boy or a girl?" but rather, "Have you had any strange cravings?"

There is no end to the list of fabled cravings that a pregnant woman might have and such fables persist. In fact, if you use an internet search engine and type in "Do pregnant women eat...", one of the first suggestions in the Auto-complete list will be "Coal"!

While there are cases where pregnant women will crave non-food items, these are very rare and obviously should not be indulged. But cravings tend to be of a very normal variety and are thought to relate to hormonal, adrenal or vitamin imbalances. As such, pregnant women will usually crave foodstuffs that are sweet or salty. At their most unusual, cravings might feature a combination of unusual flavours.

The most important aspect of food cravings is to strike a balance. They can be indulged but not excessively so. In dealing with excessive cravings, it is important for you to distract your partner from these and to promote the virtues of healthier alternatives. This should be done subtly, so as to not make an issue of the craving and reinforce it. It is also important that the negative effects of over-indulgence are understood but not over-stated; weight gain can be a concern for many pregnant women and it is important not to stigmatize the issue of cravings.

Indulge cravings in moderation. Distract from over-indulgence without derision or creating an issue.

As with the issue of morning sickness, your partner may experience aversions to certain foods. If this happens, remove them from the equation and don't have them in the house. If you have to go a few months without eggs, it's a small sacrifice!

Tiredness

Some women will have abundant energy during pregnancy, while others will have erratic and spontaneous jumps between being energetic and being incredibly tired. In general, you can expect most pregnant women to be tired more frequently during pregnancy and to have less energy than usual. It is important for you to be mindful of this and try to be accommodating and proactive.

For example, you can:

Help more around the house, leaving your pregnant partner with the minimum to do.

Plan shopping excursions more carefully to ensure that you are both getting everything you need in one visit. Try to "kill two birds with one stone" by making sure you visit the doctor and pharmacist in the same trip.

If you live outside of town, plan your necessary trips into town at times when you can find parking in areas that will minimise your time spent walking.

This next point might sound obvious but...if you do have to walk around town then plan your route to avoid unnecessary big hills! Sounds obvious, but many men don't think of these things!

Encourage your partner to rest as often as possible.

By doing these sorts of things for your partner, you will feel a more active and important part of the pregnancy. Your partner will be aware of this and as your appreciation of each other grows, so will your intimacy.

Trouble Sleeping

As pregnancy progresses, your partner may experience trouble sleeping. Your partner may not be able to get comfortable, may experience leg cramps or may need to go to the bathroom with increased regularity.

It is important not to let sleep problems get the better of your partner. Insomnia can become a vicious circle where the frustration at being unable to sleep fuels further insomnia. So, as soon as sleep problems become apparent, you should try to address them by creating a relaxing environment at bed time.

Here are some tips:

- Encourage your partner to take a relaxing bath. As well as the relaxation element, the bath can also provide your partner with respite from any backache or leg cramps that she may be experiencing.
- It is highly advisable to avoid caffeine during pregnancy as some reports suggest that caffeine can increase the chances of complications during pregnancy. In any case, caffeine intake won't help with sleep problems. It should be strictly limited and confined to day time.
- Herbal-based drinks like Camomile tea are recommended. Camomile Tea is a great remedy for insomnia. A cup of warm milk also works wonders.
- A couple of drops of Lavender Oil on her pillow are also good for a soothing effect. Lavender Oil is perfectly safe for use in this context, but it is strong so only use 1-2 drops.
- Soothing music in the bedroom before bedtime will help to set a tone for relaxation.
- Make sure the bedroom has an ambient temperature that is conducive to sleep.
- Cuddle her or give her a back rub or massage. This can create the right kind of relaxation to help her drift off.
- United we stand! If she can't sleep, stay awake with her. Again, sharing some of the hardships of pregnancy is a great way to build intimacy and convey that you will be a good father.
- Buy a comfortable pillow.

Using all (or most) of these tips as part of a routine will probably work best and be most effective.

The Bathroom

If you live in a cold climate, you should consider having a small heater installed in the bathroom if there is not one already there.

In other cases, ensure the bathroom radiator is always on or that the bathroom is at least an ambient temperature, day or night. As the pregnancy progresses, your partner will inevitably need to use the bathroom with greater frequency and at any given time, so the bathroom itself should be hospitable at all times. If you have a freezing cold bathroom, your partner may have trouble getting back to sleep after bathroom visits and the changes in temperature won't do her health any good.

Try to ensure that the bathroom is set up for your partner's convenience. Have the toilet seat down and make sure you are well stocked up on toilet roll and other essentials. These might sound like small, obvious things. But when these things are not seen to they can be a source of upset for your partner.

Also, be mindful of the need to be understanding of the problem of frequent urination. It's impact upon you is minimal compared to your partner.

The Couch

You should also be prepared to have your place in your bed usurped by a multitude of pillows as the pregnancy progresses! Some women may end up with 7 or more strategically placed pillows with them in bed by the time she had reached full term. So, bear in mind that that no matter how big your bed is, you may need to make a move elsewhere. While this isn't ideal, sleep is important for you both and this is another sacrifice that will be appreciated.

Coping With Your Partner's Mood Swings Etc.

As well as coping with morning sickness and tiredness, your partner's hormones will most likely be subject to serious fluctuations during pregnancy. This can affect her emotions in a variety of different ways and can have a more pronounced effect on some women over others. You may find that one day your partner is elated about becoming a mum, yet the next day she seems overwhelmed by what is happening. It is important to be patient and supportive of your partner throughout these swings in mood.

As Marilyn Monroe once said: "If you can't handle me when I'm at my worst, then you don't deserve me when I'm at my best!" This is especially true now, because when you show yourself to care about your pregnant partner and show an interest in how she feels, you will be building a stronger relationship that will be deeply appreciated in the better times. You will also be indicating to her that you will be a good father.

It is important to remember, too, that you realise that your partner is not instigating her own hormonal swings and is very much a slave to them too. Your partner does not want to be down or upset, she does not want to be contrary or bad-tempered. This sort of form is as difficult for her as it is for you, so don't take it all too personally.

Some tips:

Be patient, understanding and comforting to your partner. Hormones may bring tears, but there may be very real fears beneath it all and your love and attention can be the key to allaying these fears.

If there are frequent tearful episodes, it's important not to lose patience and withhold your support because you are getting fed up with the process. Your partner is unlikely to be enjoying being a slave to her hormones, so don't take it personally.

Be positive in supporting your partner. If she is having negative thoughts about the birth or motherhood, emphasise the positive aspects and don't allow her to get bogged down in negativity. Mood swings may not last long but you have to take care not to allow your partner to dwell in negativity.

Don't deride her fears as being irrational. Take care to investigate where these fears are coming from. By giving your partner adequate sympathy, this is the easiest way to determine what her fears are and how to deal with them.

Even if your partner is showing signs of emotional thinking or being irrational in her upset, ignoring it can make things worse. Whilst you may not want to over-indulge what you know to be irrational thoughts or fears, you will know from experience that these thoughts and fears pass. But failing to be attentive and supportive when she is at a low-ebb will stay with you both.

Depression affects up to 10% of pregnant women. Make sure that what you're witnessing aren't signs of depression. If you are worried about your partner's mental health then be sure to discuss this with your partner and encourage her to seek assistance in such an instance.

Coping up With Your Own Feelings

It is common, indeed to be expected, that impending fatherhood will bring with it some fear and anxieties. This is entirely natural. In fact, if you didn't experience some degree of reservation about becoming a father, then that would probably be a bigger worry! To a greater or lesser extent, all will experience feelings of anxiety, stress or fear along the road to becoming a father. Those anxieties and worries are a sign that we know how big a step we are taking, but they also show that we care about doing the right thing and being a proper father. As long as you care about the kind of father you want to become and work to make the changes that make that possible, you will be a great dad.

Here are some of the main fears and anxieties that a father-to-be will often experience.

Security: Fears about your financial situation and the security of your family are very common.

The Birth: Most men experience fears about their ability to help out and support your partner when she is in labour.

Health: You may have fears for the health of your partner and unborn child.

Relationship: It is natural to worry about how your relationship will change when there is a baby in the equation.

Personal: Men experience hormonal swings during pregnancy too! Some men can also feel detachment from partner and baby as they feel left out of the pregnancy process. There are ways to deal with these feelings.

Security

You are going to want to be able to provide the best environment possible for yourself, your partner and child. But, it is important to have a strategy in place to achieve all your goals. Otherwise, your good intentions could end up being counter-productive. Here's one example. Upon discovering that they are about to become a father, many men will enrol in college or go back to school immediately with a view to up-skilling, in order to find a better job. While this is fine and admirable in theory, many relationships end up damaged as men struggle to fulfil the new commitments they have taken on. It isn't always possible to be a part-time worker, part-time student and a full-time dad. In their bid to change their circumstances too quickly, some men will take on too much, not be around enough to lend mother the emotional support she needs and end up with less than they had hoped for.

The same can be true of men with established careers. Some will see the arrival of junior as signalling the need to climb the ladder and compete for promotions and the like. In reality, the pressure of an increased workload added to a new arrival can off-set any financial benefits for the family.

It is important to stay patient and focussed when planning for the future of your family. At the outset the most important thing you can provide is a safe, stable environment for mother and child, where mother is fully supported and baby is safe. Of course, you will need to support the family financially, but be careful not to take a blinkered view of the financial aspects of parenthood. If financial matters take priority over providing emotional support and presence, then the net outcome can be a negative.

Once you are confident that you have built a stable environment for the family, then you can discuss how best to improve you and your partner's lives going forward. Discuss the future with your partner often and be positive about it. By being positive about the future, you are far more likely to get the future you both desire and deserve.

The Birth

While the sight of men fainting in a delivery room has become something of a comedy film cliché, over three-quarters of men experience anxieties about how they will hold up when the birth happens. Many will fear becoming squeamish, panicking or passing out. In reality, it is almost unheard of for a father to pass out during labour and the vast majority of men experience very few problems with the birthing process. Much of this anxiety around birth can be directly attributed to those clichés and stereotypes of the "nerve-addled father" as depicted in movies and popular culture.

However, be sure to discuss the matter with other fathers who have been through the experience. By talking about it, you will be much better prepared for the birth when the time comes.

Health Concerns

Every pregnancy is different and they are seldom straight forward. There are bound to be little issues and incidents throughout the nine months and you are bound to have times when your fears about the pregnancy and the birth will get the better of you. However, pregnancy complications are rarer and more manageable than in days gone by and the odds of serious issues impacting on your partner and baby are small indeed.

Fears can often be nurtured by a lack of knowledge, so by becoming more knowledgeable you can allay some of these fears. Attending scans, doctor's visits and pre-natal classes are good ways to become savvier about what is going on in pregnancy.

Relationship

For some men, pregnancy can bring with it relationship anxieties. Men may feel alienated from the mother-baby bond and feel that the mother's love for her baby leaves no room for them in the relationship. It is important to see the baby as an addition to the relationship and not as a replacement for you within it.

To deal with these issues, it is important for father to bond with baby, and it is possible to do this before baby has made an appearance. Here are some things you can do to create a connection between dad and child:

Assert your role as the baby's dad. Get used to referring to the baby as "ours" and talking in terms of "we".

Attend scans so that you can see the baby's development. Many father's feel their first profound sense of connection to their child when they see junior on screen!

Learn more about when the baby is active or asleep. Ask your partner how baby reacts to a meal or how they respond to different types of music! Even if done playfully, your partner's responses will help to build your own picture of junior's personality. So, when baby makes an appearance, they won't be such a stranger!

If you can cook, ask Mum what she thinks baby would like today and cook it for them! Again, it's a playful way to include baby in activities before he/she has made an appearance and your partner will be thankful. If you can't cook, now would be a good time to learn!

Be supportive of mum and build intimacy with your partner. The more supportive and loving you are the more central to the pregnancy you become. And the more indispensable you will be!

Many relationships will come under strain when the baby arrives, as both parents may struggle with hormonal changes, tiredness and frayed nerves as you adjust to new responsibilities and an extra mouth to feed. This is the time for the greatest endurance, the most enthusiastic support and the most profound patience. By coming together during this period, you will become closely bonded and emerge on the other side as a strong, loving unit. All three of you!

Personal Worries, Anxieties and General Health

It is important that you also look after yourself during the pregnancy. Men also go through changes during pregnancy, not least of which is hormonal shifts. Studies have shown that men can experience radical changes in their own hormone levels; cortisol and testosterone concentrations may shift rapidly. Such changes are bound to impact the mood patterns of some men. In many cases, simply being alert to these changes in hormone levels can help many men to overcome the anxiety that such changes bring. After all, it is much easier to overcome an issue once you are aware there is one!

It is not uncommon for many men to exhibit symptoms very similar to morning sickness during pregnancy. This may sound strange, but as we have just mentioned, your own body is enduring a period of hormone fluctuation, so such feelings of nausea are explicable and entirely natural. In fact, shared symptoms of morning sickness may be a natural evolutionary trigger to create increased empathy between father and mother. Whatever the case, experiencing such symptoms should be seen as an opportunity to increase the empathy between you and mum.

If you continue to have anxieties or worries, don't be afraid to discuss them with your partner with a view to coming up with solutions. Also, make sure you open up to friends and other fathers. They can offer good advice and insights, and even if they don't, a problem shared is really a problem halved!

Be aware too that there are many straight forward things that you can do to be at your best and stay in a good frame of mind during the pregnancy months.

Make sure you get regular exercise. If your partner needs an afternoon rest, use this time to get out and get some fresh air. It will also do you good for your headspace. While building intimacy is important, having your own time and space is also very valuable.

Eat healthily. It can be easy to slip into a "convenience food" routine if the two of you are busy, but you should plan your meals and make sure the two of you are eating balanced diets.

Relax. There is a common misconception that people get all their regenerative requirements from sleep. This is not the case. Being busy all day and then flopping in to bed will eventually lead to fatigue. Make sure that there are periods of the day when you have nothing on and you can relax.

Meditate. No, it's not just for hippies! Meditation works and can be an invaluable source of relaxation and de-stressing. Don't knock it until you've tried it.

Growing Into The Role Of "Father-To-Be"

One really valuable tip for any Father-to-be:

If you are a passive part of the pregnancy, you will probably struggle to adjust to being a father and have trouble bonding with the baby. But if you are an active part of the pregnancy, then your transition to becoming a father will be far more manageable and far more enjoyable. And, most importantly, your bond with your son or daughter will happen more organically, more quickly and will be more solid.

The experience of becoming a father can be a stressful one for many men, as they struggle to cope with the profound change that a baby brings to their lives. In truth, we shouldn't think of fatherhood as starting at the moment of birth and if you take a proactive role in the pregnancy from the time you learn that you are to become a father, the better off you and baby will be.

Sharing the pregnancy experience with mum will take some of the burden from her and show you to be an involved and interested father. This will do an awful lot to get mum through times of doubt or depression, as she will be resolved to the fact that she is not facing into the prospect of motherhood alone. This will also do a lot to ensure that post-partum depression will not be an issue for mother, as studies show that the more involved a father is and the quicker the bond between father and baby forms, the lower the likelihood of mother suffering prolonged bouts of post-partum depression.

What You Can Do:

- Exercise with her. Whatever particular regime your partner has picked out for her pregnancy (aqua-robics, walking, swimming or whatever), by exercising with her you are doing a multitude of positive things. Exercising alone can be difficult and company can provide greater motivation, but more importantly than that, you are showing solidarity, interest and a degree of self-sacrifice that will be appreciated. You are also spending time together in which you can discuss the highlights of becoming parents or soothe any anxieties, if they exist.
- Take a pass on alcohol when you are out together. Even though you can drink, it doesn't mean you have to. By making

such a sacrifice, you are showing yourself to be selfless and considerate.

- Participate in pregnancy appointments. Scans, ante-natal classes and doctor's appointments will all reveal valuable information about the baby and about the birth. By being an active part of these classes, you will be better prepared for the birth and show yourself to be more interested and involved in the birth. Again, all these little things add up and will foster a more positive situation for baby to be born into.
- Interact with baby. Talk or read to it. Sing to it. Say hello and goodbye to it! Ask mum about the baby's activity, any patterns in movements or kicks. As mentioned earlier, if you are cooking then ask your partner what THEY would like to eat.
- Talk in WE terms when discussing the future. There will be three of you and your partner will want to hear you talking about the future with baby in mind.
- Decorate the baby's room together and participate in baby shopping. Avoid being passive in decisions regarding what the baby wears and where the baby sleeps. Express your own opinion on what YOU think baby will be into! Do so in a playful rather than forceful way, of course! But, above all, be involved.

Sex during Pregnancy from Father's to be Perspectives.

Sex will change during pregnancy for most couples. As your partner experiences profound hormonal changes, you can also expect changes in her libido. This can have radically different effects on different women, with some wanting more sex during pregnancy and others wanting less. Towards the end of pregnancy, sex may become too uncomfortable for some women, so it's important to be aware that this might happen.

It is imperative that you are sensitive to your partner's sexual needs during pregnancy and to react positively to them. Some men feel frustrated when there is less sex during pregnancy and, whilst this frustration is understandable, it is important to see the bigger picture. You, your partner and child will be together for a long time after the pregnancy, so sacrifices now are going to be worth it in the long run. Try to channel your frustrations positively into building greater intimacy between yourself and your partner during this time.

In practical terms, sex is also likely to change a lot during this time, as the progressing pregnancy necessitates changes in how you and your partner make love. This can move partners into exploring new positions that they may not have previously considered, often positively impacting their sex lives and intimacy. Indeed, couples who have been together for a very long time will admit that many of the favoured postures and positions within their sexual repertoire were discovered by necessity during pregnancy. So, far from being a limiting experience, pregnancy should be seen as a time of sexual discovery!

During Labour

Don't get caught out by the phrase "Nothing Can Prepare You For Child-birth". True, child-birth is a unique experience and until you've experienced…well, nothing can prepare you for it!

But whilst you cannot foresee what will happen as baby arrives, this is one occasion in life where being prepared is crucial. Ask yourself what your partner needs from you in this situation. Answer: A calm and supportive father. And if you know what to do, where to go, who to call, where everything is and what to expect, keeping calm will be an awful lot easier.

The more prepared you are for the birth, the more calm and supportive you will be on the day.

Squeamish?

If you happen to be squeamish about blood etc., remember, you can occupy a space within the birthing room that allows you to maximise your support for mum and minimise your exposure to body fluids and the like. Discuss this beforehand with the midwife or nurses, don't leave it until the birth when there are more pressing issues at hand. They will be helpful and will have seen plenty of people with similar issues, so they will know what works.

If you do find yourself being squeamish, bear in mind that you can use the same relaxation techniques as your partner to overcome your own symptoms. You can also execute these techniques with your partner, so that you both have a point of mutual focus during the birth.

But remember, however real and pronounced your issues surrounding the birth, they are and should remain a very distant second to your partner's needs and concerns. After all, she is the one giving birth.

TIPS FOR YOU:

- Attend Ante-Natal classes with your partner. There's no real excuse not to. They are insightful, helpful and will ensure that the birth is not such an alien experience for you.
- From the Ante-Natal classes and through research, learn about the different stages of pregnancy and become fully-versed on the labour process. By being aware of what is happening and when, you will be able to firmly establish where your partner is in the labour process. This will help you to remain calm and will improve your ability to provide your partner with assurance and support.
- Pack the labour bag around week 34 and have it left in a convenient but safe location. Ensure that you have anything in the bags is a duplicate or not necessary for everyday use

around the house...stories abound of people removing toothbrushes and the like and forgetting to put them back!

- Ring the hospital! Many first-time couples will dash to the hospital upon waters breaking, only to be sent home and told to come back later. Phone the hospital and describe the situation, the time between the contractions etc. They will advise you on what to do next.
- Know the route to the hospital. If you drive, ensure the car is in perfect working order. If you don't drive, have a designated driver arranged in advance. You might to have more than one arranged, depending on the time of day, so bear that in mind.
- Be involved. Ask questions of the nurses and midwife. Convey this information to your partner or share in its importance. Don't sit back as a passive spectator! By being proactive, you will display confidence and this will assure your partner that she is in good hands!
- Stay calm too! The best way to stay calm is to be fully aware of what the birthing scenario entails. The men who lose their composure tend to be the ones who don't know what is going on. If you have educated yourself on the process, you will be much calmer and you wouldn't be stressed by unknown phrases and unfamiliar terminology.

For Your Partner:

Interact with your partner as much as possible. Long silences may allow your partner to focus too much on the pain and perhaps allow her to drift into negative thinking.

Talk about the future; in particular, talk about after the baby is born. Talk about the clothes you have picked out and any ceremonies or celebrations you have planned. This is the reward for all you've done, so getting your partner to focus on this at the time of greatest pain will hopefully prove a distraction.

Help your wife with her breathing. Make sure her jaw doesn't clench as tension in the jaw muscles can be reflected by a contraction of the muscles in the birth canal. You can utilize Lamaze breathing techniques which are taught at most Ante-Natal classes, but one of the best breathing techniques is really simple, effective and meditative. Get your partner to repeat the word "Relax". As she says the first syllable, "Re", get her to breathe in; on the "lax" syllable, get her to breathe out. The second part is the most important part and she should breathe out as slowly as possible, extending the syllable sound as she does so and allowing all tension to leave the body. By becoming completely focussed on the word, this technique can provide valuable meditative pain relief and your partner will have a valuable distraction from her ordeal.

Massage can be of great help to your partner and your participation in it will also help you. Gentle lower back massage over acupressure points, performed in synch with breathing techniques, can provide considerable relief for mums in labour. Massage is performed on the rear pelvic region and should be a rhythmic accompaniment to mum's controlled breathing. Performing this massage early in the labour is also a great way to get directly involved from the outset and will result in much of your own anxiety dissipating.

GOLDEN TIP! If you are feeling stressed by the situation yourself, use the "Re-Lax" breathing exercise WITH your partner. This allows you to disguise your own anxiety, overcome it and in the process, by supportive and helpful to your partner without her realising you may be getting similar benefits from the exercise!

And Remember:

Take breaks at appropriate times for air, food, water and to use the toilet, preferably leaving someone close to your partner (her mother or other person permitted by the hospital) to stay with her. You need to stay hydrated and fresh. Don't stay away too long though!

As a couple, you may have had your mind set on a natural birth. If your partner changes her mind during labour, support her in the decision and be emphatic. Medical science had provided a few safe pain relief mechanisms for child birth. Use them if you need them.

The image of a father being verbally abused by his labouring partner is a bit of a comedy cliché. But, it does sometimes happen. Don't take it personally and don't let it stop you being supportive.

Breastfeeding

Breastfeeding gives baby the best possible start in life and should be encouraged. There are no real substitutes for breast milk and studies have shown that breastfeeding a child can help prevent obesity, asthma, diabetes and high blood pressure in later life.

In the more immediate term, baby is much less likely to suffer from colic, stomach upsets, coughs and colds when being breast-fed rather than bottle-fed. Babies who are breast fed are also shown to have better mental development and better dental development.

For mother, breastfeeding also has distinct advantages. Breastfeeding lessens the risk of breast or ovarian cancer, as well as reducing the risk of bone diseases such as osteoporosis. Breastfeeding will also help mum in returning to her pre-pregnancy figure.

So, with all these advantages, why do more mums not breastfeed? Well, breastfeeding can of course be very physically and emotionally demanding on mother, since she will be doing most (if not all) of the feeding of baby. Bottle feeding can seem like a convenient alternative for this reason. But remember, bottle feeding brings with it a host of time-consuming requirements. Washing bottles, sterilising and making up formula all take time. Also, most babies will go through more than one brand of formula before settling on a suitable one. And the periods when a formula is disagreeing with baby and you have to change to a different one, can be unpleasant times.

A crucial factor in the decision whether or not to breastfeed is the attitude of dad. A woman is much more likely to breastfeed if she is encouraged to do so by the father. If you are negative about breastfeeding, or even indifferent on the topic, mum is unlikely to want to breastfeed. The fact is that mum need not be so alone in feeding baby, and if you can be supportive of her and encourage breastfeeding, then you are giving your child the best possible start in life.

Some things you can do to encourage and help mum to breastfeed:

Buy a breast pump. Things don't always go to plan with regard to breast pumps and often they will go unused. Babies may prefer the breast and react negatively to suddenly being presented with a bottle, or perhaps mum will have difficulty finding enough time or milk to fill a bottle. However, if you can manage to get baby into a routine where he/she takes one bottle a day, then this could really take the edge off mum's workload and provide her with respite from the feeding process.

If you stay with mum during the feeds, this can be a great positive. If mum is feeling fatigued and breastfeeding is getting the better of her, your support can be of great help at these times. As well as this, friction can sometimes arise if mum is feeding a baby at 3am and you're snoring! While you should obviously manage your own sleep patterns and make sure you get enough sleep, be mindful of the sacrifice mum is making and try to share in it if only to lend support.

Don't make inappropriate comments or jokes. Much has been done in recent years to encourage more mums to breastfeed and to remove any social stigma surrounding breastfeeding. If mum is feeling weary from the sacrifice she's making, then inappropriate comments could undermine all this and discourage her from continuing.

Have a quiet word with naysayers and ask them to desist. It will surprise you, but within any extended group of friends or family, there will probably be one or more person who will voice disproval or who will "know better". Even if most friends are supportive, it only takes one person sharing myths, hearsay or baseless horror stories about breastfeeding to make your partner think twice. If you and your partner decide against breastfeeding, don't let it be on the basis of what others think or say.

Be supportive at every turn, but always in the knowledge that you CAN stop if everything gets too much. It's always possible to switch from breast milk to formula, but it's not possible to go the other way. If you can start by breastfeeding baby, with each passing day you are giving them a better start in life. So, be supportive and keep it up for as long as possible.

Changing Bad Habits For Fathers-To-Be

Many parents decide to give up smoking, drinking or drugs upon learning that a baby is on the way. Besides the obvious health impact that their bad habit might have upon the child, many will also be acutely aware of the financial burden that their habit causes and will see this as good a time as any to quit.

With regard to drugs, this should be seen as an absolute no-no. The risks to your child are too obvious to require explaining. Suffice to say, there aren't any examples of drug-addicted partners who have managed to provide safe and stable homes to raise their children. If you have a drug problem, you should seek help to remove the problem from your life. Many people have thought that they could "manage" a drug problem and raise a child, but none have succeeded.

If you smoke, now is a good time to quit. Failing that, there should be zero impact on the life and health of your child from smoking. So, from the get-go, ensure that you do not smoke around your pregnant partner and advise others of the same. You should smoke outside, or if the climate makes this difficult, be sure to confine smoking to a single area of the home that your partner or baby will not be frequent.

If you drink, first and foremost bear in mind that alcohol is a drug. So, the exact same rationale should apply to alcohol addiction as drug addiction. There is no place for it in your child's life.

If you are a casual drinker, ensure that you or your partner are never intoxicated around your child. Alcohol impairs judgement and impaired judgement can lead to accidents. Many people who are casual drinkers decide to keep their home alcohol-free once junior arrives. This way, they will only drink when away from junior and ensure a complete separation of child from a possible source of danger.

If you do bring drink into the home, seriously limit the quantity you allow in. There is an old Japanese proverb: "First the man takes a drink, then the drink takes a drink, then the drink takes the man." Ensure you limit the quantity of alcohol in your home to prevent such an occurrence.

And it should go without saying but, keep any form of alcohol or prescription drugs in a safe place and out of the reach of kids.

Bonding With Baby

As we have mentioned earlier, there are a multitude of ways to start creating the bond between father and baby while junior is still in utero. By implementing these tips and being more proactive in the pregnancy, you will really hit the ground running when junior appears.

By bonding with the baby early and sharing in mother's responsibilities, you are also ensuring that mother's own bond with baby develops more rapidly. When mum sees that you are bonding with baby and sharing in the responsibilities, she will be more relaxed and will ease into her own role.

The easiest way to bond with baby is to begin by simply continuing on the things you were doing while baby was in the womb. Talk to baby in the manner you've grown accustomed to, sing to baby the songs you have been singing for the past several months. Continue doing the things you have been doing and expand on these. Here are some tips:

If mum is breastfeeding, stay awake with her for late night feeds. This will show your interest, your solidarity and your desire to bond with junior. If mum isn't breastfeeding, then you should be doing your share of the feeding late at night. This will help in bond building.

Change nappies (diapers) and give the baby baths. This takes the pressure off your partner and is an important part of bonding. Some babies give their first smile while they have their nappy off and are able to kick their legs in the open air. The more nappies you change, the better your chances of being around for such a moment!

Allow baby to sleep on your belly. The closeness will increase your bond.

If possible, take some time off work in the early stages infanthood. This will allow you to help mum and to bond with baby. The more you are involved and taking the burden off mother, the greater her affinity with you grows and the stronger her own bond with baby becomes. It's the gift that keeps on giving!

In doing all of these things, you are creating a much great bond between ALL THREE of you. You are also doing much to prevent certain negative post-partum situations from developing, such as Post-partum depression. Whilst post-partum depression can be largely seen as hormonal in nature, you can do much to treat it by taking away factors that can exacerbate it or prolong it. If mum is down, here lot is worsened by the burden she bears. If you can take some of that burden, you will do much to help her overcome any lingering depression.

By being involved in an egalitarian manner, you will also prevent baby becoming a perceived barrier in your relationship with your partner. When your bonds with baby grow together, baby becomes an integral part of your lives and your relationship much more quickly.

Post-Partum Sex

You will have sex again! We say that because, in the post-partum stage, it can take a while to get back to normal and there can be a fear that "the love has gone" from the relationship if things aren't happening. But, as with many other aspects of the pregnancy experience that we have already covered, patience is central to getting your sex life back on track.

Couples often ask for a recommendation on "how long" after birth they should wait to begin having sex again. There is no straight answer to this question, as every birth is different and results in a different set of circumstances for mum and dad. It will take about 4-6 weeks for cervical closure and post-partum bleeding to no longer be an issue for most mothers. Of course, these are just the physical matters and the emotional concerns are far more important. It is only when these are addressed that you can begin to have sex again.

Post-partum sex can become an issue as the couple begins to worry that their sex life is over forever because things "don't feel the same". In reality, things simply aren't the same at first. Your partner has just given birth and feeling sexy after birth is often difficult for obvious reasons. And this is one of the reasons that things cannot be rushed.

Men, too, may often feel put off sex after witnessing childbirth. If this is the case, it is important to normalise your feelings by drifting slowly back into a situation of intimacy without rushing the sexual element. Whether it is you, your partner or both of you who feel put off, it's important not to become focussed on the negative imagery or experiences from the labour. By re-establishing non-sexual intimacy with your partner, any negativity you may have can be diffused because you and your partner will be focussing on positives within your relationship. You will likely find that, after a certain amount of time has passed, the positives in having sex again will far outweigh the negatives! And you can both return to a normal love life.

Some tips:

Couples often ask themselves the question "Will we ever have sex again?" Remember: You will!

Manage the issue by not letting it become one. Don't allow yourselves to be too focussed on it. Particularly if your partner has had a difficult birth. Thoughts of having sex may cause your partner anxiety at first. If you sense this is the case, don't press the issue. All you will be doing is raising your partner's anxiety level and pushing the return to normality further into the distance.

If it doesn't feel right, then don't do it. Amid fears that they need to do something to reignite their relationship, some couples will jump into having sex that they are not physically or emotionally ready for. They may see the need to "get it over with", so that it is no longer an issue. In reality, that can be an experience that is more damaging than bonding. It is a much better idea to wait and re-engage the sex life that you knew previously, rather than rushing in to having sex that is uncomfortable, painful or just unpleasant.

Concentrate on rebuilding the intimacy between you both. Take it very easy and slow. Try kissing, cuddling and massaging your partner. As you both gain pleasure from sharing these experiences, you will both be getting much closer to re-establishing a healthy and enjoyable sex life.

Keep things very gentle. Reigniting your sex life doesn't mean you can instantly go back to where you left off. You will probably need to have sex in certain positions by necessity before you can move things up gear. The first few occasions of love making may be a little awkward, but if your love making begins as an organic transition from acts of intimacy, such awkwardness is largely diffused. In other words, if you go from cuddling to massaging to sex and back to massaging, you won't be so focussed on the quality of the sex. And each time you have sex, it will get better and better.

While you don't want to be pushy, you should definitely let your partner know that you want to have sex with her again! Your partner may feel unsexy after being through labour and it is important for you to let her know that she is still attractive to you. So the key is to let her know this without being pushy.

If you have your own issues about having sex post-partum, discuss them with a friend other than your partner. While your issues are real and need to be addressed, you may not be helping your partner to get over her own anxieties if you burden her with yours. In fact, you may reinforce those anxieties.

Remember, many couples have felt the way you feel after the birth. Things can be strange and things can take time to get back to normal. But, they do. And the two key elements in helping you find the path back to normality are exhibiting patience and fostering intimacy.

Glossary of Terms

Acupuncture – a system of complementary medicine that involves pricking the skin or tissues with needles. It is used to treat illnesses and pains.

Acupressure – treatment of symptoms by applying pressure with the fingers to specific pressure points on the body.

Amniotic fluid – the fluid within the sac that surrounds the baby in utero

Aromatherapy -the use of aromatic plant extracts and essential oils in healing (massage or baths).

Bloody show – the passage of a small amount of blood or blood-tinged mucus through the vagina near the end of pregnancy.

Bonding – the natural attachment that develops between parents and child.

Braxton Hicks contraction – non-progressive contractions that feel like menstrual cramps.

Body awareness- being conscious of the body feelings and senses.

Breath awareness –the practice of consciously directing the breath.

Cervix – the neckline opening of the uterus.

Caesarean section – a surgical procedure to deliver a baby through the opening in the abdominal wall.

Colostrum – the first milk secreted by the breast after giving birth.

Consciousness -the state of being conscious.

Contraction – the shortening or thickening of a muscle.

Crowning- the appearance of the baby's head at the opening of vagina during delivery.

Dilation – the opening of the cervix in labour.

Effacement – the softening and thinning of the cervix.

Epidural – a regional aesthetic that is administered into a spinal space in the lower back.

Episiotomy – an incision made at the back of the vaginal opening to surgically widen the birth passage.

Failure to progress – the condition in which labour contractions are inadequate to move the baby toward delivery.

Forceps – two spoon-shaped instruments that are applied to the sides of a baby's head to assist in the delivery process.

Herpes – an infectious disease cause herpes virus.

IV drip – intravenous infusion given to a woman for different medical reasons (ex. prevent dehydration).

Mantra – a commonly repeated word or phrase.

Mindfulness – the practice of paying attention in a particular way: on purpose, in the present moment, and non-judgmentally.

Natural birth – delivery of a baby without the use of medications.

Nesting urge – a sudden burst of energy or desire to prepare for the baby's arrival that may occur in late pregnancy.

Oxytocin – a hormone secreted by the posterior pituitary gland (trade name Pitocin); stimulates contractions of the uterus and ejection of milk. Also it is considered to be a love (or attachment) hormone as it is produced during touching, kissing and hugging.

Pelvic floor – the muscular base of the abdomen, attached to the pelvis.

Perineal massage – the practice of massaging a pregnant woman's perineum around the vagina in preparation for childbirth.

Perineum – the space surrounding the vagina and the rectum.

Placenta- A flattened circular organ in the uterus which function is to nourish and maintain the foetus through the umbilical cord.

Prolapse- the moving out of space or falling of an internal organ.

Progressive Relaxation Technique – a meditation technique for combating tension and anxiety by systematically tensing and relaxing muscle groups.

Rupture of membranes – breaking the amniotic fluids membrane that surrounds the foetus.

Self-massage – when you massage your own body yourself.

Stage 1 labour – the time period from the onset of labour until the cervix fully dilates.

Stage 2 labour – the time period from full cervical dilation until the baby is delivered.

Stage 3 labour-the time period after the baby is delivered until the delivery of the placenta.

Timing of contractions – the time between the beginning of the one contraction to the beginning of the next.

Transition – the stage of labour when the cervix is nearing full dilation and contractions are intense and occurring closer together.

Trimester- a period of three month within a pregnancy.

Umbilical cord – A flexible cord like structure containing blood vessels and attaching a foetus to the placenta during pregnancy.

Vacuum extraction – using an instrument that attaches by suction to the baby's scalp to help deliver the baby.

Water birth – a birth in which the mother spends the final stages of labour in a birthing pool, with delivery taking place in the water (usually).

Suggested Reading

Practical books.

Susan Warhus, M.D., an obstetrician based in Scottsdale, Arizona. *Countdown to Baby: Answers to the 100 Most Asked Questions about Pregnancy and Childbirth.* This book provides straightforward answers to the questions Dr. Warhus most commonly received while caring for her patients.

Sheila Kitzinger, *Complete Book of Pregnancy and Childbirth. This is a* guide to pregnancy and childbirth that provides all the information women need to know in order to make decisions about prenatal tests, pain control, and how and where to give birth, with advice on the development of the foetus, body changes, and labour preparation techniques.

Jeanine Cox, *The Perfect Name.* This book provides 20,000 name possibilities and great naming exercises to inspire and educate expectant parents.

Sheila Kitzinger, *The New Pregnancy And Childbirth.* This book will inspire, inform and reassure you regarding everything from conception to birth. What to expect during pregnancy? How to prepare yourself for the physical changes ahead? Topics include Caesarean births, the birthing sling, sex during pregnancy and nutrition.

Thomas Verny, MD with John Kelly, *The Secret Life of the Unborn Child*. This book shows that the way you respond to and care for your unborn child may affect his physical and emotional well-being for the rest of his life.

David Chamberlain, *The Mind of Your Newborn Baby*. This book demonstrate that newborns are fully cognitive human beings with the ability to discriminate and experience the world in sophisticated ways.

Grantly Dick Read, *Childbirth Without Fear*. Dick-Read believed that there was something wrong in the practice of delivering babies with emphasis placed on intervention and the use of anaesthetics. He questioned whether the nature of labour was responsible for the emotional state of the women, or was the emotional state of the woman to a large extent responsible for the nature of the labour.

Humor.

Vicki Iovine, *The Girlfriends' Guide to Pregnancy*. This newly revised and updated edition, regarding these little things that are too strange or embarrassing to ask, full of practical tips, and hilarious takes on everything related to pregnancy.

Cynthia Copeland, *The Diaper Diaries: The Real Poop on a New Mom's First Year*. This is about first year of motherhood, from the hospital stay to baby's first birthday and contemplating the unimaginable-having another. There are lists, quizzes, timelines, charts, and real-life stories.

Jenny McCarthy, *Belly Laughs: The Naked Truth about Pregnancy and Childbirth*. This is a must-read comic relief for anyone who is pregnant, who has ever been pregnant, is trying to get pregnant, or, indeed, has ever been born! A very funny book about pregnancy!

For fathers.

Armin Brott's, *The Expectant Father: Facts, Tips and Advice for Dads-To-Be*. This book is not just about Brott's advice, but professional insight from obstetricians, psychologists, and sociologists regarding the changes women undergo while expecting a baby.

Thomas Hill, *What to Expect When Your Wife is Expanding*. This best-selling parody humorously guides fathers-to-be through nine months of 21st-century baby preparations. Complete with weird baby names, tips on how to avoid a sympathetic pregnancy, and much more.

Organisations

Association of Prenatal and Perinatal Psychology and Health (APPPAH)
  www.birthpsychology.com

Attachment Parenting International
  www.attachmentparenting.org

National Association of Childbearing Centres (NACC)
  www.birthcenters.org

International MotherBaby Childbirth Organization
  www.imbci.org

International Childbirth Education Association
  www.icea.org

Childbirth dot org - Where Childbirth Meets Your Life
  www.childbirth.org